The journey i
mental health h

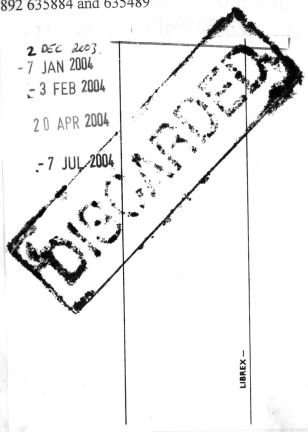

The journey in becoming a mental health nurse

Matthew V Morrissey

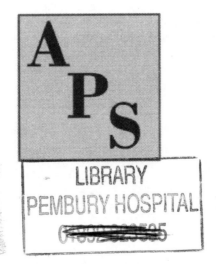

WM 100.1

APS Publishing
The Old School, Tollard Royal, Salisbury, Wiltshire, SP5 5PW
www.apspublishing.co.uk

British Library Cataloguing in Publication Data
A catalogue record for this book is available from the British
Library

© APS Publishing 2003
ISBN 0 9537234 5 3

Contents

Acknowledgements

The author would like to extend his warmest thanks to all the mental health nursing students involved who gave so freely and enthusiastically of their time. Special thanks also to colleagues, Edward Sivarajah, Andrew Thomas, Martin Arnold, Stuart Goodall, Clare Barber, Mark Wilbourn and The Canterbury Users Forum. A special thanks to groups A7, S8 and S9 for their total commitment to the project. Thanks to Valery Marston at APS Publishing for her patience, kindness and support. Special thanks to Delia Gill, Aran Islands, Co. Galway, Ireland for her encouragement and friendship. Special thanks to Barbara, Stephanie and Chris Wilson, Nick and Analeigh Chatfield, Caroline, Mark and James Duffy, Dypna Creane, Susan Bishop. I would also like to thank my family, my parents, Matt and Mary, and also Alan and Iris, Lesley, Mads, Dom and especially my son James, and Tina who is always in my thoughts.

Love and Hope

I may fall
Apart
cry
Lose it all
again
restart
my mind
it doesn't work
Let me run away
and hide
there is
no hope
for me
on any side

sitting all alone
I know
I've gained a stone
feeling agitated
my shoes are worn
I'll have a cigarette
I hesitate
I'm tortured by my brain
Can't think straight
medication again
strangers on all sides
nothing of my own
a psychiatric ward
not like home
lucid in the morning
cripples me inside
desperate for love
coldness on all sides
I get so sad for mother
She tries to be
so cool
But I've seen
Her crying
On the ward
She was so proud
Of me at school
Lost inside the system

Acknowledgements

Living by their rules
My life has little meaning
I have nothing unlike you
And you joke about the nutters
You rush around the room
But stop and think about me
I'm not so different from you

I'm nineteen with good A levels
Smart and always fun
It wasn't my plan
To be always on the run

You see I love music
And friendship
And want all the things I had
But mental illness takes them all away
I try not to be too sad

I love my brother so much
Though he doesn't understand
Although the pain I have is so strange
Being such a broken man

Its silly to want a girlfriend
Or someone to understand
But the cross is harder on your own
I'm not the same young man

When mother leaves
Or David goes
It breaks my heart to say
That sometimes I fall to pieces
Just trying to get through each day

If all I have are moments
Then make them stay
For love and hope is all I have
to get me through today

(Morrissey, 2002)

Preface

Hope, what is it? And what would be the quality of each life without it? At various times everyone needs a shoulder to cry on, but, more importantly, someone to listen and genuinely care. For those who experience or support a person with a mental health problem, hope is essential. Like carers, mental health nurses often infuse and instill hope in others so they can forge a path that can be walked together. The path of hope is well worn by both nurses, carers and users, and is made of many components, love, encouragement, reassurance, strength, tears, fear, a pair of arms and many layers of encouragement, humour and time.

Mental healthcare needs to be about people with people. It ranges from care for children to older adults. Care needs to be about the provision and protection of everyday human rights. It is a concern needing local, national and international support. It touches many people's lives, the personal and professional, politics, work, education and is explored in television and film. On a practical level, student nurses want to know what they are letting themselves in for when they sign up for a course to become a mental health nurse. Having a text that gives insights from other students already undertaking a course, or recently qualified, in mental health nursing will be invaluable. When I started to write this book, I had very little idea of the direction in which to go. The students led the way. The book endeavours to examine and discover students' experiences of becoming a mental health nurse. Interviews and short questionnaires were employed to provide the basic background. From the outset, the eyes of experience are combined with a rational and novel approach to discovering what it's like to become a mental health nurse. It is hoped that this book will be interesting, informative and an easy read for students. It is also hoped that such a text will be useful to clinicians and managers who are very much an instrumental part of the experience and process.

Introduction

'We are just walking into the dark, we don't know what to expect.'

(Keith Rusike, Student Nurse, Year 2)

The journey in becoming a mental health nurse has been, to a large extent, unchartered territory. What is the journey really like for a student? Some students come straight from school; others are mature students with vast experience. For those unfamiliar with this skilled but challenging area of work, such a question may seem redundant. Indeed, the majority of texts fail to grasp the very nature of being with people, or the comforting of those with mental health problems. In healthcare and academic courses, there continues to be a pervasive focus on science, disease and disorder. Such a focus can underestimate the power of more social methods, which could engage a person to learn and grow. However, the greatest failure is to presume that mental health nurses have no knowledge or skills.

It is important to mark out the process of becoming a person, as well as becoming a skilled and knowledgeable mental health nurse. It would be naive from the outset not to be aware of the political nature of mental health issues and the often inaccurate and confusing press, frequently linking images of violence to mental illness (Philo *et al*, 1994). Mental health is the land of milk and honey where ideas are concerned. However, when your attention is turned to practice, to the ward, to a person who is a user of mental health services, such discussions seem sadly limited.

Case study

Marion, a rather dishevelled looking lady, spends much of her day smoking cigarettes and refuses any services. Marion is one of the many glaring obstacles to medical treatment and care in the community.

As a professional, you may attend yet another conference on the brain and genetics that uncovers ever more facts, despite these often being removed from the reality faced in practice by mental health nurses during day-to-day care. The impact and complexity of mental health problems means teachers need to be not just equipped with knowledge, but must also find ways to deliver it.

Students have to contend with competing demands on their time. They need to embrace relationships that will equip them for effective practice and need general and specific information about the course they decide to follow. Unfortunately, there is very little material to draw on when students request information about what it is like to become a mental health nurse. Such paucity in the literature has serious implications for education and practice, given the need to guide potential and existing students. It is important that relevant information is available that will encourage them to consider such a career in the first place. It is clear that becoming a mental health nurse will be different from one country to another, depending on the emphasis of training, education and cultural ethos.

What is emerging is how crucial it is to understand mental health nursing students' experience (Granskar *et al*, 2001; Morrissey, in press), and to prepare them adequately with relevant supportive and constructive supervision (Morrissey, in press).

Creative and skilled mental health nurses are sculpted, developed and created, not produced. Presently, in the UK, there are many changes in and outside of the NHS that make it timely to examine student nurses' experiences, given the new approaches to curriculum, training, contracting (Sainsbury, 2002) and practice. The key concerns relate to current training and education methods and the demands and reality of working in practice.

To the general public, mental health and mental health nursing conjures up all sorts of images. Such media images are powerful and many are inaccurate, frightening and negative. For example, the film 'One Flew Over the Cuckoo's Nest' not only creates images of the darkest side of the human psyche, but also encapsulates a deep seated stereotyping of mental illness, which is cruel for those struck down with enduring mental health problems, such as schizophrenia (Morrissey, 1999). Indeed, psychiatry itself often encourages and maintains such stereotypes in a system that is disempowering and often lacking in resources for users (Heyman, 1995).

Professional ignorance continues to be a source of disempowerment for people with mental health problems, and this includes negative professional attitudes in and outside of nursing. Perhaps a more worrying facet of the nursing profession is the continued maintenance of negative and oppressive views of members of their own profession towards mental health nurses. Such negativity echoes a longstanding, oppressive, and often ignorant attitude towards mental health. Patients with mental health problems will continue to be treated either inhumanely or not the same as others while such negative attitudes go unchallenged.

Concern about the future of mental health services, and the education and training of mental health nurses, is relevant and current, nationally and internationally. It is my view that mental health nursing has as much to do with human rights as health and care. Contrary to many people's perceptions, mental health problems are commonplace, and more and more younger adults and children are affected (Nolen-Hoeksema, 2001). The enigma for many professionals us is the intense human suffering observed not only in the clients in hospitals, but also in our homes and communities.

This book will examine the experiences of several groups of student nurses who later qualify in mental health nursing. Student nurses were recruited for a research study and they identify the journey in becoming a mental health nurse. Key questions addressed by the author were related to:

- motivation to become a mental health nurse
- the ups and downs
- personal and professional lives

- what should be incorporated and considered for future curricula.

As a result, some of the nuts and bolts of what it takes to become a mental health nurse are identified from qualitative data and interviews, one year post qualifying. Snapshots are used to engage the reader and to be informative and interesting. Several models will be discussed in relation to learning therapeutic skills in mental health nursing, which is at the basis of learning (Benner, 1994). Mental health nursing is engaging, yet often challenging in both the course of study and the demands of practice.

Experiential learning is an essential tool to personal and professional development in becoming a mental health nurse. The majority of texts on mental health nursing to date are written, primarily, from a theoretical viewpoint not from a student's perspective of doing.

Knowledge is essential to tackle ignorance. The lack of relevant clinical experience would reduce learning to a simple set of outcomes. Without some structure for learning, many students would become disinterested. Learning is a continuum like learning a piece of music. To simply learn a set of outcomes about bike riding will never teach you to ride a bike. You need the experience, or at least a simulation of some kind. The environment of care for users and staff is often unsuitable. In the context of care, the architecture of the place and the people is important. This is critical if you consider that many mental health and emotional problems can often be eased by adequately-staffed, pleasant, soothing environments. To engage in experiential learning, you must be prepared to challenge your own beliefs and values, develop as a person, and grow from your own and others experiences.

Aim

The text aims to explore the process of becoming a mental health nurse from a research perspective in order to identify the process of learning for practice, and how it can be enhanced. The text will also will provide valuable insights for educationalists, clinical supervisors, mentors, managers, and students thinking about becoming mental health nurses. It is a book, which views the education and training of mental health nurses as a process of 'learning by doing', with the experience of practice as a central and focal point.

References

Benner P (1994) *Interpretive Phenomenology Embodiment, Caring and Ethics in Health and Illness*. Sage Publications, London

Granskar M, Edberg AK, Fridlund B (2001) Nursing student's experience of their first professional encounter with people having mental disorders. *J Psychiatr Ment Health Nurs* 8: 249–56

Heyman B (1995) *Researching User Perspectives on Community Healthcare*. Chapman and Hall, London

Morrissey M (1999) Fellow feelings... a mother's story of caring for her son diagnosed with schizophrenia. *Nurs Times* 95(21): 38–39

Morrissey M (In press) Becoming a mental health nurse: a qualitative study. *Int J Psychiatr Nurs Res*

Nolen-Hoeksema S (2001) *Abnormal Psychology*, 2nd edn. McGraw Hill, Boston

Philo G, Secker J, Platt S, Hendersen L, McLaughlin G, Burnside J (1994) The impact of the mass media on public images of mental illness: media content and audience belief. *Health Educ J* 53: 271–81

Sainsbury (2002) *Briefing Paper 16: Acute Inpatient Care for People with Mental Health Problems*. Sainsbury Centre for Mental Health, London

1

Our knowledge is caring: A brief history of mental health nursing

'To us the ashes of our ancestors are sacred and their resting place is hallowed ground'.
Chief Seattle, Chief of the Dwamish,
upon surrendering his land to Governor Isaac Stevens in 1855
(cited In: McLuchan, 1993)

The history of American Indian culture is fascinating and holds a special place in the hearts of many people in understanding the value and connectedness of all living things. It also shows that history is not just recorded on a page or in a book; it can be living and alive. In particular, there is a strong oral tradition in the Indian culture. This tradition is very much part of mental health nursing culture. Historically, Indians fought many battles and were always under threat from the white man. It seems mental health nursing has been, and is still, dominated by the medical model in relation to care, is bound in medical power, ritual and rules, and has had to survive a number of attacks and criticisms. More than this, mental health nursing has been pulled in different directions by the medical model, different and often conflicting therapeutic approaches from psychoanalysis to behaviourism. However, mental health nurses, too, can find their own voice by reclaiming what is rightfully theirs throughout history—the knowledge of caring for people with mental health problems.

Men and women who become mental health nurses need to value and respect people in the past who have lived and died for the relief of human suffering. There must also be an appreciation for the suffering of people with the mental health problems that exists today. Underlying the history of mental health nursing is awareness and respect that gives meaning to people's lives. It is important to respect the knowledge and skills of professionals, teachers, users and carers. We can also learn much from the history and wisdom of other cultures, however alien they may, at first, appear.

> 'The man who sat on the ground in his tipi meditating on life and its meaning, accepting the kinship of all creatures and acknowledging unity with the Universe of things was infusing into his being the true essence of civilization, and when native men left off this form of development, his humanization was retarded in growth'.

Chief Luther Standing Bear

In the history of medicine and psychiatry, it seems knowledge not caring is power. Throughout the history of psychiatry, there is almost an obsession with knowledge, cure, treatment and ownership. Medical knowledge is only one form of knowledge, but, as we are now discovering, the knowledge of caring needs to be reclaimed in order to value mental health nurses as people, including valuing their knowledge and skills. In the past, our teachers have handed down many things, but the greatest of these must be respect for human life. Respecting the fact that each person has a history is a very important first step.

In mental health nursing, the knowledge of caring can be person-centred, intelligent, precise, respectful, well executed and can be done with ease, if the person has knowledge and is skilled. However, if all you see is the surface, you may be under the illusion that such behaviour is without knowledge or skill. Wisdom comes with appreciating the purpose and result of reasoned action.

The knowledge of caring is clearly a solid foundation for mental health nursing, now and in the past. However, what patients sought and needed then, and users seek now, is not just medical knowledge, but the knowledge and delivery of sensitive care. This knowledge, which has been handed down throughout history, is one method of reclaiming our past. This knowledge of caring in mental health is primarily a nursing concern, and the use of specific skills of caring separates mental health nursing from other disciplines, including that of medicine. Nurses are much more of an authority on caring, as they assess deliver and monitor the majority of hands on care.

In this chapter, it will be shown that mental health nurses, caring for people with acute and enduring mental health problems, are not just an addition to psychiatrists. Mental health nurses are now challenging the lack of caring instilled by a purely medical model. Nurses deserve more than token respect for their work and expertise.

It is evident that research and clinical work around caring practices needs a much higher priority and investment. Mental health nursing, or psychiatric nursing, has its own history with a developing body of knowledge and skills concerning caring for users of mental health services. This includes developing ongoing support and education for families, based on care not cure. In the world of multidisciplinary care, this ought to give nurses a certain respect, power and kudos. We need to redefine and reclaim what is rightfully ours, the fundamental right to care with respect and dignity, to give users real choices. To become masters of hope for users of mental health services and their families, we must mark out our territory carefully before it is eroded.

It will be argued that, in order to execute a suitable standard of care, we must learn to reinstate, reward and demonstrate a respect for the knowledge and wisdom of caring mental health nurses. Historically, mental health nurses have been in the presence of users, which means they observed many forms of mental and emotional distress and real hardship. Part of this approach is to respect nurses' important contribution to the everyday lives of users, carers and and other colleagues, such as nursing assistants. We need to build a new science, based on sharing and promoting good care practices, in the knowledge that nurses are strong together. We can develop and promote a new mental health nursing—the science of caring—only if caring is valued, well resourced, effectively managed, practice- and research-based, and takes place in a purpose built environment.

Introduction

Contrary to popular belief, many students are interested in stories from the past and enjoy looking at photos, videos and films that can bring past events to life. If one could sit on the edge of time and watch how people with mental health problems have been, and continue to be, treated, we may be much more conscious of our own lack of humanity and the need for compassionate care. There are many ideas surrounding mental healthcare, yet it is high quality nursing, psychological and medical care that continue to be rare commodities.

Unlike medicine, which has many artefacts, our history requires astute detective work in putting together facts, and these should include anecdotal accounts. Our history as mental health nurses is important to our identity, as it helps us to understand past and present processes of care. It also outlines where we have been, where we are now, and possible directions for the future.

History

One of the earliest beliefs held that a person with a mental disorder was possessed by demons or evil spirits; this was initially espoused by the ancient Egyptians, Chinese and Hebrews (Veith, 1965). Exorcism employed methods, such as prayer, magic and the use of purgatives concocted from herbs. If these failed, more extreme methods were taken to ensure that the body would be an unpleasant dwelling place for evil spirits. Flogging, starvation, burning and even stoning to death were not infrequent forms of 'treatment' (Atkinson *et al*, 2000).

The first real progress in properly understanding mental disorders was made by the Greek physician, Hippocrates, (circa 460–377 BC.), who rejected demonology and maintained that mental disorder was the result of an imbalance in body fluids. Hippocrates, and the Greek and Roman physicians who followed, argued for a more humane treatment of the mentally ill. In particular, they stressed the need for pleasant surroundings, proper diet, massage and soothing baths, as well as less desirable treatments, such as bleeding, purging and mechanical restraints (Veith, 1965). Later, punishing the mentally ill was associated with punishing the devil, and cruel and barbaric treatments ensued. Witchcraft saw thousands sentenced to death during the fifteen, sixteen and seventeenth centuries (Kroll, 1973). This history is part of the background to the development of the history of medicine, psychiatry and nursing.

Modern discourse

What good is the history if it only gives one microcosmic view? Historically, mental health nurses, like users, were subsumed into a lesser or an unimportant category (Nolan, 1993) as shown in social research by Goffman (1961). Yet, in reality, many of the changes in care for users were fuelled and implemented by the mental health nurse. At best, nurses are portrayed in history as hand maidens to doctors, under their control and in the shadows of an oppressive and damaging culture. Such a culture was cruel and lacking basic humanity (Selling, 1940).

In medical and psychiatric history, there are always promises of new cures, and in the fantasy, the focus diverts to fairy tale attitudes and sadly unrealistic expectations. Often, at the end is a drug which has uncomfortable side effects and fails to cure. Beyond this is a person, a user, in some cases needing protracted care and support, and the learning of new coping skills. Mental health nurses work with individual people not a diagnosis or a disorder, and our history binds us to users more than any other professional. Most other professionals visit acute wards as consultants of one kind or another. Yet these consultants are not responsible or very much involved in the hands on delivery of care. Nurses are in the same environment as users for the most significant amount of time and demands on their time are often intense and multidimensional.

Nurses continue to be the armoury in hospital and community mental health services that deliver care, reflecting the past and present roles. Hands on care has been our domain for centuries and, whatever medicine may have thought in the past, we are now an educated workforce with our own developing knowledge and skills.

Historically, there have been many cruel and barbaric treatments of the mentally ill, often delivered by the orders of medical madhouse proprietors (Burrows, 1828). Indeed, medical men who owned and ran most of the madhouses wanted to outlaw the lay madhouse keepers. Many physicians stated openly that the treatment was superior in madhouses kept by medical men. They claimed that medical madhouses offered a cure, while those of lay madhouses only offered custody.

Such a claim was false scientifically and is a fallacy even now, as psychiatry fails to cure the majority of common mental health problems, for example, schizophrenia. There are real difficulties controlling symptoms in many disorders and causes remain elusive. Sometimes physicians even fail to accurately diagnose for many years (Hill *et al*, 1996). The notion of cure is, perhaps, a sign of early arrogance and hunger for power in medicine and psychiatry. Of more concern is that it throws out the notion of care as less important. Currently, it is the view of many that some issues in mental health are best seen outside a medical or illness framework, particularly for users (Heyman, 1995).

Knowing what was done to innocent people in the past causes feelings of intense shame, injustice and pain. To walk through some of the large institutions, now empty, reawakens the sound of haunting and terrifying voices of the past, fear permeating the boarded windows, now a nesting site for birds others becoming modern housing developments. It identifies the dramatic speed of change within our current history framework. It takes a very special eye to see that, if we are not careful, history may repeat itself and come back to haunt us.

Indeed, in a relatively short time some changes, such as the generic work (Anonymous, 2000) may erode the very relationships and roles that have carved the term 'mental health nurse'. More than at any other time, we must work together to recognise the special value of each person, including our colleagues; for each person leaves a history.

It is not good enough just to prevent cruelty to animals and children. People with mental health problems are frequently at risk and cared for more and more by untrained staff with little education or experience. Just being adequately fed and watered should not be considered the hallmark of modern mental health or elderly care services. Nurses only spend a fraction of their time in therapeutic relationships (Sullivan, 1998). History is reticent about historical asylum care, and current practices in psychiatry can still reflect some of the negative and barbaric past.

Lack of appreciation of the past tends to foster over evaluation of modern achievements and the assumption, so stultifying to progress, that what is present is good and what is past is bad (Hunter and Macalpine, 1970: 3). This is such a valuable insight given the many visions that have never been realised in science, psychiatry or mental health nursing.

It is surprising that any intelligent person could have anything but respect for caring mental health nurses. Today, nursing students who choose to be mental health nurses are intrinsically our living and unfolding history. They can bring boundless energy, humour, sensitivity, enthusiasm, care and excitement to courses in mental health nursing. This is a challenge to those of us involved in shaping and providing courses in this important field of knowledge and practice.

User movements

By recognising the success and the strength of the user movement in the UK, it becomes evident that any future courses must include these voices to give relevant information a more user-centred approach (Morrissey, 1997; Wood and Wilson-Barnett, 1999). It is important to bring the voice of users into mental health nursing programmes. Users are the focus of our history. They are the reason we exist and listening attentively to users reminds us of what it takes to become a mental health nurse. This is not just from an academic viewpoint, but also involves caring from the heart and sometimes the pit of our stomach .

In practice is where we learn about human dignity, the amazing stories of the courage of users, a recognition of the pain individuals and families go through, often behind closed doors, and the deepest level of respect for their needs. It remains important to foster hope if care is to have any chance of success.

Our history binds us to some of the most important aspects of humanity and compassion. Mental health nursing needs to be bound in the protection and promotion of human rights and not rest simply on theoretical or academic concepts. Like users, mental health nurses frequently have to fight for basic resources. It should never be presumed that atrocities in mental healthcare from the past are gone forever and could not happen again. Indeed, even a cursory glance at suicide figures would suggest otherwise (Nordentoft *et al*, 2002). An examination of a brief history of the mental health nurse seems a useful place to begin our journey into the process of becoming a mental health nurse.

A brief history of mental health nursing

To advocate the power of mental health nursing, we must not be afraid of reclaiming what is rightfully ours; namely, our history. We need to reclaim our knowledge of caring, and its clear link with mental health nursing as protection for human rights, and our solidarity in providing care not cure throughout history. This can be achieved by a close and careful examination of the past, skimming our way through various accounts and artefacts, patching our history together. To examine the journey of becoming a mental health nurse, it is important for students to briefly explore where we have been, where we are now, and where are we going. In the current demands of practice, it is important to learn and gain insights from the past to effectively underpin the future developments in mental health nursing.

Recent histories of psychiatry indicate that history is not just about the well sung heroes, but is also about the middle and lower ranks who are often sanitized, not seen as important or ignored. The history of psychiatry is only one aspect of the history of mental healthcare (Leiba, 2001; Nolan, 1993) and is often focussed on medical achievements, which have not always stood the test of time or science. What is clear is that those left to care for people who were mentally ill were often uneducated and unskilled. Could we go this way again? It is clear that nurses have never had the resources to execute a fraction of the skills they posses and there is little indication that they ever will unless real resources are put in place.

In the eighteenth and early nineteenth century, those who looked after the mentally ill were referred to as 'keepers'. In 1845, the term 'attendant' emerged and female attendants were referred to as 'nurses'. It was not until the end of the nineteenth century that the term 'nurse' became neutral, either male or female. In 1923, the term 'mental nurse' became the official title and later in the 1940s the term 'psychiatric nurse' was adopted. Mental heath nursing in Britain towards the end of the last two decades of the twentieth century employs four different terms interchangeably: 'mental nurse', 'psychiatric nurse', 'nurse therapist' and 'mental health nurse'. The terms 'mental health nurse' and 'psychiatric nurse' are the most commonly used today in journals and in practice. A review of the literature surrounding the history of British nursing suggest that, at best, psychiatric nursing has been considered an appendage of either general nursing or medicine and, at worst, an irrelevance, meriting little or no acknowledgement in the history of care (Nolan, 1993).

The rise of the anti-psychiatry movement in the 1960s, was led by figures, such as Szasz, Laing, Sedwick and, most notably, Foucault, who, over time, challenged psychiatry in its view that psychiatric care was predominantly their history alone. Since Foucault, nurses have been empowered to ask why they have only been allocated a very marginal role in the pages of history despite having had the most intimate therapeutic role in relation to the mentally ill (Nolan, 1993). In fact, while psychiatry was, and often still is, about confinement, nursing is about building bridges and fostering and promoting hope. Historically, little seems to be known about the practices of mental health nurses in the past. It is time to reclaim what is rightfully ours—the knowledge and skills of caring.

A summary of some key dates and events

Where we have been: The Middle Ages

1148: Earliest charitable hospital St Bartholomew's Smithfields, London

The first mention of care worker was Master, who was required to visit, comfort and confer the sacraments of the church. Monks, also called basket men because they collected alms, were superintendents when connected to a monastery. Other names used at this time were keeper or rector. Punishment inflicted on inmates and staff consisted of: flogging, fines, fasting, suspensions and expulsions. Mentally ill patients were admitted to the same houses as those with physical diseases and not accommodated in different wards.

1247: House of Bethlem Founded by Simon Fitzmary

Bridewells' houses of correction workers called beadles

1312: Distinction between lunatics and idiots; protection of their estates de Praerogative Regis of 1312

This is perhaps the first mental health legislation (Edwards, 1975).

Sixteenth and seventeenth centuries

Men segregated from women in care, routine, power, surveillance, and discipline, and rules for day-to-day activities dominated.

1537: The Order of the Hospitals of Henry VIII

The keepers were to be virtuous, responsible for management, reporting faults and punishments (Russell, 1997). Male keepers were generally recruited from farm servants and females from domestic servants. Physical strength and sobriety were generally enough. Treatment consisted of bleeding, purgatives or emetics. Chains, belts, locks, belts, cribs secured with chains, irregular meals, lack of exercise, abusive remarks, degrading names, beatings, and blows with fist or straps or keys was a daily experience of patients' everyday existence. The status of the keeper was that of a lowly servant (O' Donaghue, 1914).

1601: The Poor Law

This law made it possible for county justices to oversee the inmates well-being. These people were from then on in the custody of keepers, beadles in Bridewells and madhouses (Leiba, 2001).

Seventeenth and eighteenth centuries

Physicians became central figure in confinement to what became known as the trade in lunacy. By the end of the eighteenth century, the physician had manipulated confinement into a medical space, yet at that time, medicine was just a re-invention of the old rites of order, authority, discipline and punishment. The emergence of the private madhouse and those in charge varied from doctors and clergy to quacks and laymen.

1788: Responsibility by medicine for the insane was slow and protracted, but the selection of the Reverend Dr Willis to treat King George III in 1788 was an event of great historical importance, as it brought some respect to the trade in lunacy. It showed that treatment of insanity required special skills not possessed by even the most skilled physicians. At this time, there was a fight for the lucrative trade in lunacy and the medical men owned most of the madhouses and tried to outlaw lay madhouse keepers. They considered their treatment superior and curative.

1813: Tuke at the York Retreat argues for the principle of moral restraint.

1828: Burrows highlighted the cure versus lay view, which was presented to the Select Committee of the House of Lords.

1860: The official policy stated by the Commissioners was not to issue licences other than to medical proprietors. Medical men then owned many madhouses simultaneously, residing in none and, of course, leaving the work to servants, superintendents, keepers and attendants. In the early nineteenth century, attendants were involved in care and in the move from custodial duties and the use of mechanical restraint to employing the technique of moral restraint put forward by Tuke .

The asylum

Some of the best and most vivid descriptions of institutional and asylum care is provided by the writings of Irving Goffman (1961). At this point in history, the title 'attendant' replaced the title 'keeper' who watched and experienced first hand the development of the asylum system. Asylums were governed by rigid, often autocratic, rules and discipline. Inmates were used for labour and, towards the end of the nineteenth century, there was rapid expansion in industries within asylums and hospital grounds. Wages were very low and conditions were often appalling, so criteria for recruitment was frequently very modest. Physical restraint was supposed to be used as a last resort, moral restraint being used instead (Leiba, 2001; Nolan, 1993).

In 1837, Brown had called for some system of instruction for attendants. However, it was not until between 1842 and 1844 that Sir Alexander Morrison gave the first set of lectures specifically to attendants at the Surrey Asylum. More lectures followed in 1854, but it was not until 1871 that Henry Maudsley proposed that the Medico-Psychological Association set up a registry of good attendants; sadly, he failed to link this to any form of training. Training did follow some time later and examination papers were set by the Medico-Psychological Association. In 1885, a book was published, *A Handbook for Attendants of the Insane.*The training led to a certificate for attendants, most of the training being provided by doctors and included massage and first aid.

In the middle of the nineteenth century, the asylum system took charge of care and treatment of the insane. They exercised control rather than cure. In 1845, the Lunatics Act clearly helped blur the distinction between discretely mental and physical disorder. The Act included the protection of the insane against illegal detention and the involvement of social workers. The 1890 Lunacy Act was developed in a social climate that grew in its critical view of services available to the insane. Attendants training was considered inferior to general nurse training and there was intense opposition in trying to unite training for attendants provided by the Medico-Psychological Association and the Royal British Nursing Association. In 1895, the resolution was adopted and moves were also adopted to bring mental nursing in line with other forms of nursing. However, many years passed until 1919 when it was finally sealed by the Registration Act for England, Scotland and Wales. Mental nurse became the official title in 1923 (Nolan, 1993), although it was probably in use before this. However, it was not until 1943 that the now well known Royal College of Nursing accepted that mental nurses should be dually qualified as general nurses, and not until 1951 that training for mental nurses had passed entirely into the hands of the General Nursing Council.

Becoming modern: mental health nursing

The Mental Treatment Act of 1930 tried to identify mental illness as being similar to a physical illness in the belief that it would reduce or eradicate the stigma of mental illness.There were marked changes in terminology; asylums to hospitals and inmates to patients. There were enthusiastic attempts to cure mental illness, which introduced the intensive use of insulin therapy, electro-convulsive therapy, psychosurgery and drug therapy. This cure ethos included treatments that were familiar in horror movies, such as padded cells, strait jackets, forced feeding, etc. The nurses were trained on the implementation and monitoring of the new cure culture, which was dominated by medical treatment. Alongside this, nurses were expected to attend to the hygiene of the ward, and this included sharing chores, such as polishing floors, with patients.

In 1959, the Mental Health Act was published and came into force, and nurses were involved in implementing physical restraint and the maintenance of institutional life. At the same time, community care was developing, thus enabling the development of community psychiatric nursing. The 1959 Act was instrumental in extending the role of the mental health nurse to working in the community, as patients were discharged to their homes, health centres and outpatient clinics. The introduction of psychotropic drugs to treat mental disorder might have contributed to de-skilling nurses (Hunter, 1956). In 1966, The Salmon Report (DHSS, 1966) on nursing management structure created a new role, the nursing officer, primarily a management and supervisory role.

There has never been any research published into evaluating the role of nursing officers or their impact on nursing practice. Many issues arose in the sixties about concerns for care of the mentally ill and many letters were written to newspapers about the dreadful conditions of hospitals at that time (Robb, 1967). In 1983 came another Mental Health Act, which moved treatment into civil rights for patients. The Mental Health Act Commission was set up to ensure good practice with respect to consent to treatment, and second opinions were implemented correctly. Social workers were more involved in admission.

The Jay Report (DHSS, 1979) focussed on the change in emphasis to more psychological models of care, and nurses were seen to be central to therapeutic work, adopting a role as therapist. The syllabus now presented mental health nursing as very different from general nursing in its theory and approach. However, ten years later, this was radically undermined with the introduction of Project 2000, which again tried to identify the similarities between all nursing and the institution of a Common Foundation Programme. Mental health nursing has been dogged by the dominance of medicine, legislation and various paradigm shifts that have significantly changed and reduced the role and development of mental nurses.

As a result, nurses tend to place less emphasis on inter-personal and social knowledge and skills, and are implement-ing a much more clinical and biologically-based approach to care. There are more and more reports stressing the need for social and psychological care and the protection of the person with a mental health problem and, increasingly, the public (Dept of Health, 1996; Dept of Health, 1995).

There are serious implications for nurses in relation to surveillance after discharge, follow up and treatment in the community. Such roles are exemplified in the Mental Health Patients in the Community Act 1995 (Dept of Health, 1995). There is a clear indication that supervised aftercare is possibly a resurgence of the trade in lunacy, with the nurse continuing to be the subordinate. It is clear that for others it may be seen as a return to the dominance of the medical somatic approach to the care and treatment of the mentally ill (Leiba, 2001). If this is true, we are likely to see an increase in litigation and an increased need for vigilance in protecting the rights of the vulnerable.

Where are we now; what's in a name?

Today, it is not uncommon to hear children or adults call each other a nutcase, a nutter, etc, and indeed it is quite common in today's society for the word mad to mean interesting rather than mentally ill. Being a bit crazy is almost a sign of a positive and vibrant personality, particularly where creativity and artistic temperaments are concerned. In the Middle Ages, those involved directly in caring for people who were often termed insane, lunatic, crazy, nutters, basket cases, idiots, etc, have a long and protracted history and a number of titles from master to nurse. If you examine many historical accounts and texts, you will find that there are numerous associations with clergy and priests and often a priest was responsible for the care of the insane in special institutional settings. It is clear that men were at the forefront of much of the caring work (Brown *et al*, 2000).

Historically, knowledge of care is clearly fuelled by nurses not doctors. This is in keeping with the strong history that mental health nurses have in the protection of human rights. Attendants observed many of the atrocities and later acted as a stronger moral conscience, finding their own way to appease suffering and protect lunatics from the cruelty of others. It is perhaps noteworthy that therapeutic skills and care in mental health as we know them today may have been developed on the backs, knowledge and skills of attendants.

In the medical literature, it is clear that some doctors advocated better conditions for attendants and nurses. Dr Kirkbride valued highly the asylum attendants and his views were esteemed by others. Because of his considerable reputation, his writings on attendants are a focal point in relation to developments in care at that time. In 1841, he prepared a manual for attendants in which he spelt out the requirements of a 'good attendant':

> 'A high moral character, a good education, strict temperance, kind and respectful manners, a cheerful and forbearing temper, with calmness under irritation, industry, zeal and watchfulness in the discharge of duty and, above all, sympathy which springs from the heart, are among the qualities which are desirable'.

(Tuke, 1884)

Having a history is vital and creates the foundation of the service provided, and lessons from the past and other nursing authors support this view (Leiba, 2001; Nolan, 1993;). Understanding of our past reinforces the ability to be informed by the past and lays the building blocks for future approaches to practice. For many students today, part of this recognition is in developing and understanding their own personal and professional identity as mental health nurses.

Mental health nursing history is very much subsumed by the history of psychiatry. Much of the history has been delivered by retired psychiatrists who have had particular messages to convey to a particular audience whose interest in mental health nursing was minimal and satisfied by the most casual allusions to nurses (Nolan, 1993). The majority of these historians have tended to see nursing as an integral part of psychiatry, with no separate existence from it.

The total picture is a medical picture lacking any real focus on the value of the work of nurses. It may be that the reluctance felt by psychiatric/mental health nurses to examine their history is due to a feeling of what they will find or uncover. Many attempts to document the history and development of the mental health nurse have, to a large extent, focussed on nursing as a female career.

From historical accounts, nursing achievements should not be confined to viewing nursing as a female occupation; this is a myth. Men are no longer put off by sexual stereotyping and view nursing as a profession, identifying positive role models on television programmes, such as 'Casualty, and one in ten nurses are now men, compared with 1 in a 100, fifty years ago (Dail Mail, 2002)

Recently, it has been suggested that men have been at the forefront of caring work for centuries and it was not until the mid nineteenth century, when shifts in the nature of masculinity and femininity occurred (spearheaded by Florence Nightingale), that nursing became feminised (Brown *et al*, 2000). In specific areas, before and after the asylum, care was primarily delivered by men. It is clear that the nursing profession must draw on the past accurately to underpin current and future practice. Men and women have their respective places in history, but this must also be expressed in nursing practice and society as a whole.

Recruitment remains an issue in the UK (Doult and Stephen, 1998) and Ireland where reasons are far from clear (Wells and McElwee, 2000). However, keeping an eye on the development of generic staff is important as this could erode the specialist skill and knowledge of the mental health nurse. This may be a retrograde step, presuming that all skills are transferable and all knowledge the same.

Recent reports, like Sainsbury (1997; 1998; 2001; 2002), highlight the changing roles and the pace of change for mental health staff and, more specifically, the implementation of The Capable Practitioner, Care Programme Approach and the National Service Framework (DoH, 2001; Sainsbury, 2002).

There are a number of concerns, but the most critical is that nurses should not be used as just a pair of hands for other professionals' perceptions of change. Throughout history, mental health nurses have struggled against the odds. It seems that, in order to implement any major change in services, those on the ground need to be strategically involved. As yet there is little evidence that the strength of mental health nurses as catalysts for change has been fully explored and valued. Of more concern is the increase in the number of people working with the mentally ill, who have very little experience and often no knowledge or training in mental health. Such a state is reminiscent of the distant past and to some extent things seem worse, not better, supported by some reports (Sainsbury, 1998). The consequence could lead to poorer practices, infrequent monitoring and a reduced quality of care.

Currently, there is a need to focus on a critical review of nursing and psychiatry, and allied health professionals in mental healthcare to identify key issues in the UK, drawing on specific health reports and legislation. Mental health services need to be carefully planned and no amount of legislation and policies will meet the needs of poorly resourced services. From the outset, students must become aware of the new, emerging and broader picture of mental health in the UK and must be encouraged to take their part and use their voice in discussions surrounding the issues for users and services. Part of this must be an awareness of the work of the user movement. It is now evident that there is much positive strength in collaboration, and the fostering of smaller self-help groups. (Lelliott *et al*, 2001)

If nurses are to be any real part of a plan for mental healthcare, key nursing resources and strategies of the workforce must be identified and strengthened. This also impacts on nurse education, the environments of care, and practice preparation of student nurses at university to make sure they are adequately prepared for practice. This is important given the changes already being implemented in mental health services and primary care.

It is possible that the achievements and abilities of mental health nurses to lead services will be undermined, if their knowledge and skills are viewed as generic or less capable than other practitioners, such as doctors, psychologists or social workers. Ironically, UK nurses are more educated than ever before, yet there are still barriers to delivering effective multi-professional education and observable and measurable multi-disciplinary practice.

It is vital to appreciate that images of mental health nursing in the past and present are often shrouded in ignorance. Education and understanding is required in helping students to develop knowledge and understanding. Such knowledge can only be gained through continued exposure, positive and constructive experiences, education and clinical support. When we have reclaimed our history, we can take pride in the terms 'mental health nurse', or 'psychiatric nurse' in the knowledge that our history predates medicine and has outlived science.

References

Anonymous (2000) Generic staff will change mental health nursing. *Nurs Stand* **14**(45): 9

Atkinson RL, Atkinson RC, Smith EE, Bem DJ, Nolen Hoeksema S (2000) *Hilgards' Introduction to Psychology*, 13th edn. Harcourt, Fort Worth

Brown B, Nolan P, Crawford P (2000) Men in nursing: ambivalence in care, gender and masculinity. *Int Hist Nurs J* **5**(3): 4–13

Burrows GM (1828) *Commentaries on the Causes of Insanity*. Underwood, London

Daily Mail (2002) *Men in Nursing*. October 30th: 18

Department of Health (2002) *Acute Solutions*. HMSO, London

Department of Health (2001) *The National Service Framework for Mental Health*. HMSO, London

Department of Health (1996) *The Spectrum of Care: Local Services for People with Mental Health Problems*. HMSO, London

Department of Health (1995) *The Mental Health Patients in the Community Act*. HMSO, London

Department of Health and Social Security (1979) *Report of the Committee of Enquiry into Mental Handicap Nursing* (The Jay Report). HMSO, London

Department of Health and Social Security (1966) *The Report of the Committee on Senior Nurse Staffing Structure* (The Salmon Report). HMSO, London

Doult B, Stephen H (1998) Recruitment drive for mental health nurses. *Nurs Stand* 13(12): 5

Edwards AH (1975) *Mental Health Services*. Shaw, London

Goffman E (1961) *Asylums: Essays on the Social Situations of Mental Patients and Other Inmates*. Penguin Books, London

Heyman B (1995) *Researching User Perspectives on Community Healthcare*. Chapman and Hall, London

Hill RG, Hardy P, Shepherd G (1996) *Perspectives on Manic Depression; A Survey of the Manic Depression Fellowship*. The Sainsbury Centre for Mental Health, London

Hunter R (1956) The rise and fall of mental nursing in the mental hospital. *Lancet* July 14: 98–99

Hunter R, Macalpine I (1970) *Three Hundred Years of Psychiatry 1535–1860*. Castle Publishing, New York

Kroll J (1973) A reappraisal of psychiatry in the Middle Ages. *Arch Gen Psychiatry* 29: 276–83

Leiba T (2001) An introduction to the history of mental health nursing. Cited in: Forster S, ed. *The Role of the Mental Health Nurse*. Nelson Thornes, Cheltenham

Lelliott P, Beevor A, Hogman G, et al (2001) Carers' and users' expectations of services—User version (CUES-U): a new instrument to measure the experience of users of mental health services. *Br J Psychiatry* 179: 67–72

McLuchan TC (1993) *Touch the Earth: A Self-portrait of Indian Existence*. Abacus, London

Morrissey MV (1997) A survey of information provision in mental health: what have we learned? *Int J Psychiatr Nurs Res* 3(3): 361–69

Nolan P (1993) *A History of Mental Health Nursing*. Chapman and Hall, London

Nordentoft M, Jeppersen P, Abel M, *et al* (2002) OPUS study: suicidal behaviour, suicidal ideation, and hopelessness among patients with first episode psychosis: One-year follow up of a randomised controlled trial. *Br J Psychiatry* **181**(43): S98–S106

O' Donaghue EC (1914) *The Story of Bethlem Hospital from its Foundation in 1247*. T Fisher Unwin, London

Robb B, ed. (1967) *Sans Everything: A Case to Answer*. Nelson, London

Russell D (1997) *Scenes from Bedlam*. Balliere Tindall, London

Sainsbury (2002) *Briefing Paper 16: Acute Inpatient Care for People with Mental Health Problems*. Sainsbury Centre for Mental Health, London

Sainsbury (2001) *The Capable Practitioner*. Sainsbury Centre for Mental Health, London

Sainsbury (1998) *Briefing Paper 4: Acute Problems: A Survey of the Quality of Care in Acute Psychiatric Wards*. Sainsbury Centre for Mental Health, London: 20

Sainsbury (1997) *Pulling Together: The Future Roles and Training of Mental Health Staff*. Sainsbury Centre for Mental Health, London

Selling LH (1940) *Men Against Madness*. Greenberg, New York

Sullivan P (1998) Therapeutic interaction in mental health nursing. *Nurs Stand* **12**(45): 39–42

Tuke S (1884) On the mental conditions in hypnotism. *J Ment Sci* **29**: 55

Veith I (1965) *Hysteria: The History of a Disease*. University of Chicago Press, Chicago, IL

Wells JSG, McElwee CN (2000) The recruitment crisis in nursing: placing Irish nursing in context: a review. *J Adv Nurs* **32**(1): 10–8

Wood J, Wilson-Barnett J (1999) The influence of user involvement on the learning of mental health nursing students. *Nurs Times Res* **4**(4): 257–70

2

Forever the new boy or girl: Becoming a mental health nurse:

This chapter employs a qualitative research study of the experiences of student nurses in order to consider the process involved in becoming a mental health nurse. It attempts to describe, connect, discuss, and understand the process of becoming a mental health nurse in theory and practice using a qualitative approach (Burnard, 1991; Field and Morse, 1994; Glaser and Strauss, 1967; Hammersley, 1992; Holliday, 2002). A questionnaire and semi-structured interviews were used to examine the student nurses experiences prior, and one year in, to their first staff nurse post. The terms 'psychiatric nurse' and 'mental health nurse' continue to be used interchangeably in practice and in written texts. However, for simplicity, the term 'mental health nurse' is used for this text.

'You can do it. Just try...now you see you can do it. Well done!'

Although such comments are not written into any curriculum, it is so important to encourage and find ways for students to develop new skills and knowledge. Surgeons, nurses, and artists learn their craft and skills by observation, modelling and doing. Users of mental health services also need continual encouragement, yet it is so easy to forget the difficulties they face .

'I couldn't rest so agitated all I could do was cry, I felt like the angels had abandoned me, so fragile like a baby, led into a world of disturbed people, praying that it was a bad dream begging my family not to leave me. I saw my mother crying and I was going mad inside crying all the time, I was sure that my boyfriend would leave me—Marie the nurse was my only comfort my only hope.'

(User)

'It can be a lonely journey at times, It's the unknown, leaving one group and joining another to start the mental health branch. I'm not sure what to expect, but I am glad to get to this point as that is why I came here in the first place. It's difficult leaving my CFP group (Common Foundation Programme) and I am nervous...I'll miss my friends'.

(Student, Year 3)

While new drugs in mental health are a major industry and seem very exciting, there is growing concern among nurses for the care crisis in mental health, nationally and internationally. The fabric of much of this care is provided by mental health nurses. Yet to date, the medical profession dominates, as do the enduring mental health problems they claim to cure. In contrast, nurses continue to care for these individuals and, like users and their families, are increasingly aware of the limitations of pharmacological and medical interventions. Contrary to the myths about people with mental health problems, there is, as yet, no drug that provides high quality care or cure. Until science can be certain of the underlying mechanisms for the elusive cure for major mental health problems, emphasis needs to shift in developing effective nursing and social care, early intervention, and specific healthcare that needs to include primary and daycare facilities. A vital aspect of care is provided by mental health nurses.

Despite anecdotal accounts, mental health nurses are valued enormously by users of mental health services not only for what they do, but for their relationship with users (Hill *et al*, 1996). However, the process of becoming a mental health nurse is rather less researched or understood. It is timely for other professionals and funding bodies to begin to value the very special care and vital contribution to people's lives that skilled mental health nurses can make. The journey in becoming a mental health nurse takes three years, but many say you only really become a mental health nurse after qualifying. Students say this is, in part, to do with a sense of being responsible and dealing with real issues in dynamic and diverse situations. More importantly, the hands on aspects of clinical practice define what the nurse needs to know to do the job.

Whatever the experience of students, the education of mental health nurses in the UK is now firmly based within a university setting. Nurses on clinical placements work either in the community or in a hospital setting. Few professionals would argue that the two cultures are very different. Here is where the student's story begins. Interestingly, like junior doctors, some students take to practice more readily than theory, no matter how it is dressed or delivered. Some have quite negative views of classroom learning, particularly if it represents past difficulty or failings.

You have to really live the plethora of experiences as a student nurse and personal tutor to fully appreciate the journey in becoming a mental health nurse. Some students have mountains to climb in coming to terms with their experiences and dealing with their own issues. Others have a natural gift with people. Many need to learn to take care of themselves. There may be difficult questions to answer and the answers only generate further questions. In mental health, we have to figure many things out for ourselves, making decisions and taking responsibility for our actions. Part of the process means questioning and comparing approaches to the same issue or problem. Students learn that qualified staff, including psychiatrists, live within boundaries of knowing and not knowing. Mental illness is complex and diverse, and has many grey areas. Starting as a student is sometimes difficult and more so if you are a long way from your family.

> 'It was lonely and scary at the start I missed my family...especially my small sister...on my first placement... I will always remember Karen. She was more like a nurse to me than a patient.... I was so very scared... I think as you get more experience, confidence comes with that.'

> (Student, Year 1)

> 'Looking back as a student, you are always on the move. The placements are only a few weeks and you never get your foot under the table; you are always meeting new staff. It's hard to fit

in, it really isn't easy, it's frustrating, you are forever the new boy or girl.'

(Student, Year 3)

'Sometimes staff won't let you do certain aspects of care, yet on your previous placement you were doing the same things unsupervised, it's frustrating and makes no sense'.

(Student, Year 2)

'I'm just an ordinary 19 year old, a bit shy. I remember I was nervous at the interview and was asked mainly about why I wanted to be a nurse and my previous experience. I was glad I prepared for the interview. Although I was quite positive about the outcome, I didn't really relax until I had the letter of confirmation'.

(Student, Year 1)

'I really struggle with essays and things. I didn't come to write essays, I came to be a nurse. I never liked school so I guess I'm struggling a bit, but I really love the work with patients'.

(Student, Year 1)

Introduction

Unlike a geography student, a nursing student is about becoming a health professional, being responsible or at least assuming some responsibility as an adult for the care of others. More than this, students have to juggle work life, academic work and personal life, and develop a professional personae. Such an emphasis hardly makes the university experience carefree days. They begin in the classroom, then undertake a clinical placement, before returning to university repeatedly over the three year course. This in itself creates fear for and can be quite daunting, especially if you are the person on the seat. It is remarkable is how well most students adapt to the demands.

At some point in their nursing course, each student has to make an important career decision about the branch of nursing in which to specialise, i.e., child, mental health or adult nursing. Those with experience can decide beforehand, while others suffer a real dilemma in making such a decision.

Literature

In the literature, there continues to be much debate surrounding mental health nursing (Altshul, 1972; Barker, 1999; Gournay, 1995; Regel and Roberts, 2002; Sainsbury, 2002; Watkins, 2001). Alongside this debate, there is now an increasing need to focus on the learning needs and experiences of student nurses in practice. Mental health nursing has been described as primarily a skills-based profession (Peplau, 1987) and this was clearly evident within the 1982 training syllabus, which prescribed a skills based curriculum. Indeed, there remains the question for some as to whether there is sufficient understanding as yet of what a skill is in relation to mental health care, and what is a skilful nurse (Gijbels, 1995; Nolan, 1993)?

Much of the literature tends to be quite prescriptive about what the nurse should do (Brooking *et al*, 1992; Gijbels, 1995). Burnard (1989) claims that we still do not know what mental health nursing skills are, or what skills are therapeutic. However, more recent publications suggest the opposite, based on evidence from current practice (Gamble and Brennan, 2001; Watkins, 2001). It is more accurate to state that mental health nurses have a range of expertise, knowledge, and skills, and some are clearly advanced and expert in their field.

Many studies have also identified barriers to effective mental health nursing in practice over the years (Altshul, 1972; Carr, 1979; Sainsbury, 2002; Sainsbury, 1998). In summary, ideological differences, inter-professional conflicts, administrative duties, educational deficiencies, bureaucratic constraints, organisational structures, personal inabilities and unwillingness, low status, environmental unsuitability and managerial pressures have all been identified to explain why nurses do not perform as promoted in the prescriptive literature (Gijbels, 1995).

A more recent Swedish nursing study examined student nurses' experience of their first professional encounter with people with a mental disorder (Granskar *et al*, 2001). The findings of this study will be discussed later in relation to becoming a mental health nurse, which is the focus of this book.

In this present study, readers will be drawn to the fact that students experience becoming a mental health nurse in very different ways and, for some, the journey is a total redirection of their nursing career. It is clearly evident that mental health nurses place a great deal of emphasis on relationships, interpersonal communication, rapport, therapy, relaxation, experience, knowledge and skills.

If a good rapport is developed from the start, nursing students engender enthusiasm, fun and new ideas about nursing and mental health. They can offer important human insights and experiences with respect to the theory and practice of mental health nursing, and bring vitality, a freshness to the subject and joy to the lives of many clients while they are on placement. Their input is incredibly valued by many qualified nurses and the author. This research is an exciting partnership between teacher and students who aim to learn what it is like and what it takes to become a mental health nurse from the voice of students themselves. The research study below will discuss the process of becoming a mental health nurse.

The study

The impetus for this study, and subsequent book, developed because of the students' need for insight into what it is like to become a mental health nurse and work in the field. Students helped to design much of the content. In part, the study and book aim to lay basic foundations that will help students gain an insight, even before they start their nursing course. The study was descriptive and employed a qualitative approach, using a questionnaire and semi-structured interviews.

A volunteer sample of 68 student nurses was drawn from three different cohorts of students over one year. The draw back of such a method is that the sample is self-selected, with only those who are willing, participating. This may give a distorted view of the topic. Sandelowski (1986) refers to this as a form of 'elite bias'. For the same reason, it is important to find respondents with knowledge of the topic under investigation (Holliday, 2002).

Data

Data was gathered using a questionnaire and in-depth audio interviews with the consent of each student. The type of interview employed was a semi-structured, in-depth interview (Burnard, 1991; Hammersley, 1992) and is usual in this type of qualitative research design. The rationale for this approach to analysis was to allow respondents to give accounts of their own perceptions of their experiences, in their own words.

The transcribed interview data were analysed using thematic content analysis (Burnard, 1991), a method adapted from a variety of other research approaches (Field and Morse, 1994; Glaser and Strauss, 1967; Hammersley, 1992). The purpose of this method of analysis was to draw meaningful relationships in the data and to develop a systematic investigation of the themes, connecting these under a detailed and exhaustive category system.

Themes

The themes and categories that emerged were related to the questions asked, and through independent raters (Burnard, 1991; Hammersley, 1992) and also to the author's knowledge and understanding of the topic being researched. Content analysis implies the expectation that meaningful patterns exist in communication. However, its significance cannot be assumed only by virtue of its categorisation.

Findings

Seven categories were identified: client-centred nursing-style, observation and listening, fear, knowing/not knowing, becoming..., use of self and interpersonal skills, job satisfaction, and mastering hope. An interesting place to start exploring the experience of students was to discover how they decided to follow a path in mental health nursing.

1. Client-centred nursing style

The data suggested that one of the primary reasons students choose to do mental health nursing concerned working more directly and independently with clients and, in particular, the style of nursing interaction. Some students changed direction altogether, as a result of their negative experiences in general nursing.

Why did you want to be a mental health nurse? (MHN)

'Because when I did my sampling experience in mental health, I really enjoyed it. Originally I never wanted to be a mental health nurse I wanted to be a general nurse. The main reason was because I had worked in nursing homes and care in the community. I never really imagined for one minute that I would become a mental health nurse. I wanted to do general and then when I got to work on the general side I hated it.

I hated it because you never really got to know the patients. It was always so and so and patients wanted to talk. But, sometimes they would have no one to talk to and you were never available because you were being told to do some other non-important task; it was never about getting to know someone. For example, if someone was upset or crying and you could see that they were really miserable, you could never do anything about it and you were told to leave them on their own.'

(Female, 26-year-old student; Year 1)

Mental health nursing students find it difficult to nurse when the client is not the centre of care. This is important, as the focus of much of the work of being a mental health nurse is believed to be about relationships. In mental health nursing, the nurse is seen as a facilitator, not necessarily the lead or an authority figure (Peplau, 1987; Watkins, 2001). It is not unusual for a student to rethink his/her original career in adult nursing and decide to follow mental health nursing. This is often as a result of a clinical placement.

'Then I started reading their notes and then gradually realised that perhaps that this was more my type of nursing because they can get closer to care. Whereas in general nursing I didn't like the way they talked to the patients and that was it really. I did my general and detested it. I think mental health nursing is for people who want to think and general nursing is more for people who want to do'.

(Male, 31-year-old student)

'I made the decision to do mental health nursing from the start. It was always mental health nursing. I had no aspirations to be a general nurse at all. I'd worked with patients with mental health problems for a long time and enjoyed working with patients and I decided to do my training as a means of furthering my education and moving my career on, really.'

(Female, 32-year-old student)

'I liked the uniform to start with...[laugh]. I didn't actually want to be an MHN to start with. I really didn't want to go into that field at all. In fact, I remember contesting quite strongly when they wanted me to sample mental health, and I was allocated an acute ward at that.

When I first started, they said that they couldn't guarantee that I would see anything, but within the first half hour all hell broke loose and it was just horrendous, I couldn't believe it. I remember saying to another student, I am not coming back here again. But I think it was ignorance on my part. Really it was fear. There were a lot of highly psychotic patients there. But I decided this was the nursing career for me; I really enjoyed working closely with patients'.

(Male, 31-year-old student; Year 3)

2. Observing and listening

Listening to students is really helpful as they see things with fresh eyes. Students viewed observing and listening as important core skills in becoming a mental health nurse. For example, the section below indicates how the astute observation of a student nurse led to action in offering client care in the form of listening and support for a user, with a positive outcome. Observation is not just about behaviour, it is about monitoring emotional and psychological states, personal safety and the safety of others.

> '*I must say to hear a grown man cry...kind of makes me want to cry too... but you have to keep your cool... and well we all chat about things at handover or in a group... Michael was agitated and I knew he was getting more wound up... and well he likes me, God knows why... [laugh] so I asked him if he'd like to go for a walk and he did... he doesn't really talk... but I could see he was more relaxed when we came back...and so I think little things help. I always reassure him, especially when he feels low... I found it hard at the start... I didn't know what to say or do... you learn but its not easy ... but after a while it comes more naturally.*'

(Student; Year 3)

> '*All I did was listen to Eamon for a few minutes, that seemed to help and so each day I would just sit with him and he would talk quite naturally with just the odd nonverbal cue like nodding. It took me a while to learn these skills as I am normally very chatty.*'

(Student; Year 2)

A short walk in the right company can make a difference to a person's well-being. In reality, many acute settings do not have a garden or time to take people off the ward, even for short intervals. In contrast, many students have commented in rehabilitation settings how remarkable the rapport can be with users and how amazed they are at the ease of relationships.

Students often observe and notice little things, the important things that can make a difference to a user's well-being and often their ordinary dialogue can make a dull day bearable.

> '*We were in the kitchen... and the chat was so natural between nurses and residents... I had to pinch myself to realize I was on duty... and after a while I was able to chat myself... it was nice... the laughter... I felt part of it... I didn't know there was such places until I was on my community placement... It was so nice to be part of a rehabilitation setting...and learn the benefits of doing ordinary things... at another persons pace...*'.

(Student nurse)

It may seem strange that listening to a piece of music or sharing a joke with a user can make you realise the deep affection and respect that many users have for mental health nurses. Human bonds are so important in our work and students are moved by what they see and, of course, sometimes feel frightened. Students, like anyone else, need to feedback and discuss their placements and such insights need to be fed back to placements. As mental health nurses and students, we are placed in a key role when working with users in and outside of the hospital setting.

Students realise how brave and courageous many of the gifted young and old people are who have a mental health problem. It is obvious that they have a deep compassion for people in their care and it is not unusual for a student's comments to make staff rethink care approaches. Students are also afraid of making blunders during their education or practice. This fear might be a result of their uncertainty about acting on intuitive feelings.

3. Fear

Many students reported feeling high levels of fear about not knowing what to say or do, of the unknown, about trying to fit into the work culture and the student culture, etc. For example, many students, including mature students, are often afraid to say anything while they are on placement and need practical encouragement and support.

> 'Well you know you have your report and well you don't want to do or say anything to jeopardise that'.

(Student)

This fear could be associated with a student's need to be liked, fear of making incorrect assumptions, or not fitting in. Such feelings can undermine learning and confidence. It can raise concerns at being in an institutional setting and being placed in the position of having to respond instantly, without thinking, and to making sure that the correct forms are signed. Mental health nursing ought to be about enabling and advocating on behalf of users; yet, at times in clinical practice, fear permeates the lives of many students:

'I was scared of being hit or assaulted, I didn't know anything at the start about mental health, however, I wasn't the only one... but after the sampling placement I began to relax... I realized that these days you are more likely to be assaulted on the street...'

(Student)

At times during the course, students admitted they were afraid of the unknown, of making mistakes in practice, saying the wrong thing or being unprepared. Ironically, these are the very feelings that users have to come to terms with; for example, in relation to their diagnosis and trying to battle the stigma and negative expectations of themselves and others. Like users, students need to come to terms with the uncertainty that can be stressful in itself:

'My heart sank. I knew this would be a difficult placement, I knew a lot of things, but didn't want to share them as I didn't want to come across as a know-it-all like they said in my last placement... I was genuinely afraid to put a foot wrong... it's stressful sometimes when you don't know what is expected... and, yes, I feel more guarded now.'

(Student)

If more and more acute care is custodial, relationships might not be formed or severed, and we will end up like prison wardens rather than caring nurses. Students will feel unable to contribute ideas and new approaches. Some would say we are already there, judging from published reports (Sainsbury, 2002). Being comfortable in another person's company is a compliment and to be at ease is a hallmark of closeness and intimacy. Listening attentively to, and learning from, students helps to keep our feet firmly grounded. Currently, the demands on qualified nurses and student mental health nurses in acute settings can be physically, psychologically and emotionally draining (Sainsbury, 2001). Students are special and often bring with them, or must learn, complex people skills, astuteness, maturity and compassion to care for people with mental health problems.

Users on acute areas are often desperate for someone to listen to them and need the specialist knowledge, skills, support and help of nurses. But skills and knowledge take time to develop, so students should be encouraged to try the knowledge they are acquiring in group work as part of their education and then in practice before they care for a client. Getting to know your self should be part of the course in theory and practice—self-awareness an important first step.

4. Becoming... Use of self and interpersonal skills

In a number of ways, mental health nurses draw directly from the self (the most authentic part of who we are) in order to work with another person. Interpersonal skills, such as observation and listening to others are used to communicate and learn about others' thoughts, feelings, and behaviour. Students need to be willing to risk saying the wrong thing in order to conquer their fear of not being adequate in a given situation. This can only be achieved if trust and rapport are established and is more likely to happen if the supervisor teaches the student in practice, by example. The student needs nurturing until he or she has the necessary skills, first to survive and then to progress into therapeutic relationships.

If students interact freely with users, they can learn to utilise basic interpersonal skills to safeguard their own feelings as well as those of users. Ordinary social communication sometimes needs to be learned; not every student can engage naturally and confidently with users and colleagues. They must learn to scrutinise their own coping styles and work in a more positive way with the difficulties of others.

This is where a mentor or clinical supervisor is important and preferably should be someone the student can relate to easily and with whom he/she is able to have regular contact. However, in clinical practice, it should not be presumed that such supervisors are adequately prepared for these roles; many lack support themselves.

The use of self is the basis of effective mental health nursing, a view that is supported by many (Atschul, 1972; Peplau, 1987; Watkins, 2001). More importantly, academic, caring, interpersonal and communication skills, emotional support, integrity, confidentiality, counselling and practical skills are all being developed, simultaneously. The use of self is complex, takes time and comes by using building blocks, such as interpersonal skills. If the student can engage with a client under supervision as a novice, he/she gains feedback from the supervisor. Interpersonal and communication skills can be honed by coaching; thus the student feels he/she has progressed and the supervisor can feel confident that the student has understood the processes and is developing his/her skills. Use of self is ongoing, and most mental health nurses know that we learn from the situation and the person. Nurses may be able to work better with some clients than others, and it is not easy to know why, even from the experienced nurse's point of view. A key aspect to learning is flexibility and the growth in self awareness.

In practice, it is important to develop the skills of learning how to befriend a person with emotional or psychological problems and how to ease another's distress. To observe a student nurse engage and support someone in distress, who has twice his/her age and experience, is to witness part of the process of becoming a mental health nurse. This involves appearing calm, communicating, comforting, reassuring and being confident in dealing with such anxieties. These qualities are honed over and over by students and qualified nurses.

The 'becoming' part of mental health nursing is frequently overlooked or undervalued in the cure culture.

> 'The actual use of interpersonal skills and the fact that you have to rely on your interpersonal skills to be a mental health nurse... more than any other skills. I found the other people who worked on the wards... the qualified nurses and nursing assistants were far more approachable than general nurses. It was far easier to ask questions as a student nurse, why are you doing this, why is the patient acting in this way. They seemed like a nice bunch of people to work with on the whole'.

(Female, 22-years-old student)

These skills are important for nurses to learn and possess, and develop over time, often taking years to perfect. It is important for a user or colleague to learn the quality of the presence of a student nurse. Basic, non verbal behaviour can be demonstrative in conveying care and warmth. With the right supervision and support, the student can be relaxed in delivering care up to his/her level of competence.

5. Knowing... not knowing

A constant theme in the lives of student nurses is what they know or feel they should know and perhaps this is related to the applied or doing aspects of becoming a nurse. This may explains why some students, even though assessed and deemed to be competent, think they are not or lack confidence. Students frequently find it difficult to establish a benchmark between theory and practice. Confidence comes with mastering this fear and slowly realising their own ability to manage situations effectively.

> 'I think the more I get with my final placement the more I think there is so much I don't know. The closer I am getting, the more I worry about all the things I need to know... the other side of this is that you start to realise you know more than you thought you knew'.
> (Student, Year 3)

The experience of not knowing persisted even a year after qualifying. For new students and senior students, this differed significantly. There was a different not knowing experience for new students. New students are checking out what they have to learn and senior students are checking out whether what they have learned and know will be enough in practice as a staff nurse.

What was it like starting branch?

> 'Scary, on the first day they seem to throw everything at you, I was exhausted as I was so nervous, I'm sure nothing went in that they said.'
> (Student)

> 'Well really I felt guilty leaving my two children, and really I was more thinking how will I survive this practically, emotionally and financially'.
> (Student)

> 'I'm 50; all my friends thought I was mad, but I wanted to do it, apart from being scared... I wondered if my brain could cope... [laugh].
> (Student)

What was it like after qualifying?

'I began to realize how much I have changed as a person, people around me noticed. I became stronger and it has definitely changed my relationship with those closest to me. Sometimes I'm not sure if it is all so positive. On an acute ward you don't get much time to reflect on things and already there is so much more to learn and to deal with'.

(Student)

'I think the further I got into rostered service I realised that there is so much more I don't know. The closer I am getting to the end of my third year, I am thinking of all the things I need to know. However, on the other hand I do now realise that I know more than I thought. I can feel myself getting that bit more confident. I think it actually helps having other more junior students on the ward. You can give them confidence in turn by encouraging them letting them know they are doing the right thing. Also they give you feedback and say you handled that situation well, I wouldn't have known what to do. And later you sit back and reflect and think… God… I knew what to do without thinking about it.'

(Male, 31-year-old student; Year 3)

'Scary, very, very scary. I was the sole qualified nurse in charge of the ward three weeks after qualifying. I coped I think because of the good relationship with the nursing assistants and drawing on things I had learned. However, one year on I am far more confident now. I think one of the other things as mental health nurses is that we can ask doctors what we need. For example, I'd like the patient to have this. And a lot of the time because we don't have doctors on site, we have to phone up and ask the duty doctor. Now I have the confidence to say I need so many mgs of diazepam, which I didn't have the confidence a year ago. I wouldn't have even known what to ask for. My knowledge of drugs has increased significantly and things like section papers I found easier to grasp. We are often put under dangerous staffing levels. Being the only qualified nurse with two nursing assistants on an acute ward.'

(Female, 26-year-old student; Year 2)

Students bring many things to practice, a vibrance and a quality of hope, a fresh approach, an acceptance, giving of themselves to another, a simple but encouraging force, a little nudge to move another person to aim further and higher. Students want to try things. They love feeling that they made an impact and often give incredibly detailed feedback on the positive aspects of staff, and are very constructive about how to improve things. There are so many hurdles for students, both in theory and practice, and they are very much individuals, some with children and family commitments. They, too, have life events to deal with like boyfriend, girlfriend problems, loss, divorce, financial problems, being home sick, failing assignments and moving house. Unlike other courses, the demands on student nurses in mental health are multi-dimensional and need to be researched and understood.

6. Mastering hope

In mastering important skills, the ultimate task for the nurse is to foster hope in another human being, for without hope there is no progress. Many students talked about trying to work with people with enduring mental health problems and trying to find the right level to communicate. Some spoke about coming to terms with their own feelings and responses to events, the sadness they witnessed and also about important successes. In fostering hope, students mentioned the importance of social communication, patience, having a good sense of humour and being there for a person.

Students need to recognise that becoming a mental health nurse is the integration of knowledge and many skills, intrapersonal and interpersonal, to culminate in therapeutic relationships that foster hope. There is a need to be more secure yet transparent as a person to foster hope in others. This might come with experience and a natural propensity to care, but mostly by trust in their abilities from themselves and others. All nurses need encouragement and positive feedback, but, for some, compassion, empathy, genuineness are just words on a page.

A nurse has to draw from deep wells of inner strength and compassion to help others, and this is about taking risks. Advanced and expert mental health nursing work is knowing, using and learning about professional and personal boundaries. Respect is a key element to expert practice. Some nurses may take on roles, such as teacher, friend, or counsellor, to build alliances. Different situations demand different levels of empathy; for example, on a rehabilitation setting or in an acute psychiatric ward. Goals and feelings of achievement for nurse and client should not be underestimated. Such structure is important in terms of personal and professional development and also contributes to job satisfaction.

7. Job satisfaction

'I think you are working with patients longer and you see them achieve goals which are really good for them as a person. In mental health I find it interesting that they come in with problems and they reach for something and it's really a good thing they have achieved. And if they relapse and have to come back you remember them.'

(Student)

Many students expressed increased job satisfaction with the kind of relationships formed with clients and being able to see them progress and recover.

What do you like about being a mental health nurse?

'I enjoy what I do which has been a big plus because up until now in my career I've never enjoyed my work ever... I've just got up and gone to work. So I did the course and really enjoyed it and most of the placements.'

(Student; Year 3)

'I felt I did more for the patients, I found it more interesting than general nursing. On the adult ward I'd felt I had completed the tasks but I hadn't really helped anybody's life much.'

(Student; Year 3)

'I think when you are working with people with mental illness, you know what you see on the outside is just the tip of the iceberg.

When you actually get to know the person and discover things about them, only then do you start to find out what is going on.'

(Student; Year 3)

'I find it interesting because it's always a challenge to get to know people. I just find it really enjoyable. It's so diverse. I previously worked as a support worker before I did my nurse training and I wanted to have more of a platform because I had gone as far as I could without getting qualified. So it seemed like a natural progression.'

(Student; Year 2)

'For me, I still like to see the progression from a patient being unwell to being well again. I get a great sense of satisfaction. Teaching someone new skills, coping mechanisms, learning about their illness. It's wonderful to go from being in hospital for a long time being unwell, moving back into the community, into a flat, getting a job or returning to education. That's where my satisfaction comes from.'

(Student; Year 3)

Becoming a mental health nurse is about relationships and this is reinforced by student nurses' responses in the above extracts. But it is the way these relationships develop that sets the skills of the mental health nurse apart, moving from the known to unknown. However, it is clear to nurses on the ground, that staff shortages could have catastrophic effects to care, and this is supported by recent studies (Gournay, 2000). As a student nurse or qualified nurse, you are working with a client in a private space—another person's life. Many nurses gain much satisfaction from the closeness of being with another person and assisting them back to independence or an improved quality of life.

Being with a user of mental health services or dealing with another person's mental health or emotional problem may be daunting for some students. But clearly education and experience that builds on the abilities and strengths of each student will facilitate the development of personal and professional confidence (Morrissey, 2001). Persuading the student to give feedback on the placement is important, particularly concerning relationships. It helps students to have space to work out their own feelings and concerns. Also it is a place to ask questions and feel they can express fear or uncertainty openly. Sometimes students need to explore their fears about developing a mental health problem or of catching an illness from a person in their care.

Discussion

From the data, the motivation to become a mental health nurse tended to cluster around valuing the type of relationships with users and the autonomy of the student. Becoming a mental health nurse was important, if the person was placed as the main focus of care as opposed to being done for and to. Students in mental health nursing are more likely to view their role as being about thinking than just doing. The steps in becoming a mental health nurse seemed to come from utilising past and present experience. This included checking out what had been learned in practice, while valuing interpersonal, learning and observational skills. It appeared that these skills were honed again and again in the development of therapeutic relationships. Students recognised barriers to developing relationships in practice, such as, lack of resources, role conflict, and fear of saying or doing the wrong thing.

Being a mental health professional is different to just having a set of competencies or skills. It requires intelligence about decisions that affect people's lives and being able to prioritise. Group discussion is an important part of this process (Wilkinson and Wilkinson, 1996). Becoming a mental health nurse isn't just about a three year diploma or degree course in nursing, it involves integrating knowledge and skills in a variety of areas from law to advanced clinical practice. There is a need for structures that support continued educational and clinical progression for newly qualifying nurses.

In nursing, stigma surrounding mental health is sometimes translated into a deep seated fear or disrespect for mental health nurses, who are often viewed as 'not proper nurses' in practice and education. Such views are entrenched in nursing and such stigma is not uncommon as was recently commented on by Rabbi Julia Neuberger (ENB, 2002). This may indicate that the stigma of mental illness permeates not only lay beliefs, but also so-called professional attitudes. It is strange that nurse colleagues could have such negative attitudes given the dreadful emotional and psychological distress that many mental health nurses work with day in and day out, particularly in acute settings.

Perhaps of more concern is the environments of care, which do little to enhance the image of progress in mental health. Clinical psychologists, social workers, psychotherapists and doctors are often visitors to wards leaving nurses to provide round the clock care. It is to nurses that users and relatives turn. It is nurses who are in charge of care on our busiest acute mental health wards. It is nurses who deal with the crisis in practice.

It is important to understand the two lives of the mental health nursing student in both university and in practice settings. Clinical placements are often only eight weeks at the start of the branch programme in mental health. As a result, students often see themselves as always the new girl or boy, never settling, always on the move and never quite being accepted. Moving from one clinical placement to another means that students are forever introducing themselves to new colleagues and environments. It is, perhaps, in listening to the voices of students that progress can be made in designing new programmes in university and practice. In mental health nursing, our casualty is emotional and psychological.

At the end of the day, perhaps hope is the only thing left in services starved of resources. A recent study examined nursing students' experience of their first encounter with mental disorder (Granskar et al, 2001). Although useful, the model focusses exclusively on students' feelings in a theoretical model. Another concern is that the authors presume feelings are simple. It excludes complexities of the internal and external world, including situational variables. More than this, the sample size of 11 could hardly be considered as a representative sample. Encounters with people, including people with mental health problems, are likely to involve complex information processing that includes past experiences and complex feelings of which the student might not even be aware. Any model that aims to represent students' experiences needs to appreciate the social and psychological complexities of human experience and human interaction.

Nursing students qualities

	Focussed on their own needs	Focussed on patients' needs
Rejecting The student	FEELING HELPLESS	FEELING CONFIDENT
Establishing a relationship with the student	FEELING CONFIRMED	FEELING PROUD

Figure 2.1: Nursing students' experience of their first professional encounter with people having mental disorders (Granskar *et al*, 2001) *Theoretical Model*

Becoming a mental health nurse: Theoretical model

Moving on from first encounters with users, the study about becoming a mental health nurse identified seven main themes, or categories, from the data. The research identified that students' encounters with users draws not just on feelings, but on their past, personal and work experiences, thinking, emotional reactions to users and staff, the way they work, the environment, philosophy of care, their own knowledge, feeling of confidence and skill level. It is interesting that the category 'knowing and not knowing' meant that, even after three years, newly qualified nurses were still checking out what their knowledge base was. Perhaps, there is a tendency to make wrong assumptions about skill acquisition from first encounter to competence in practice. The main themes identified as being central to becoming a mental health nurse by students were: having a client-centred nursing-style, observation and listening, fear, knowing/not knowing, use of self and interpersonal skills, job satisfaction, and mastering hope. This can be translated into a theoretical model identifying the process of becoming a mental health nurse. The world of the student nurse becomes more complex, the more you are immersed in their world, both at university and in practice. What is clear is that the students' views of becoming a mental health nurse is quite different from actually being one. The world between being a student and being qualified is stressful, finding the right role, the right level of interaction and then receiving feedback from clinicians. Many students said they never knew if they were doing anything right, as they tend not to get positive feedback. Some wondered if there was a right way and many indicated that current staffing levels compromised learning. Skills development is an essential part of becoming a mental health nurse, which often needs considerable input from clinicians in practice, and is not always possible. A model is useful in understanding the process of how students need to learn in practice. The Therapeutic Skills Acquisition Model is represented in the model (*Figure 2.2*).

In order to learn therapeutic skills in practice, student nurses need to have an identified clinical supervisor. They also need the ability to observe good practice, have role models, be able to try out new skills, and acquire a clear idea of their competence. This requires time and energy. Like doctors, nurses need to learn by observation and doing. The link tutor can arrange meetings to ensure that learning experiences are available and that clinical supervision takes place and is monitored. A major problem for nursing is that mentors and supervisors are also delivering care and, if staffing levels are low, learning, feedback and instruction will be limited. Unlike occupational therapists and doctors, the work of mentors is not protected time in nursing and they do not get paid for it.

The learning loop identifies a starting point for each student and supervisor. Although the student may have covered the theory in the classroom, such knowledge often needs to be reactivated in practice. Coaching skills are needed by the supervisor and the link tutor, which should not be presumed because of formal qualifications. Then follows rehearsal where the student is sometimes reassured by the supervisor and in some cases by the link tutor. However, feedback is the most essential element of this process and often overlooked. The acquisition of the skill is the next stage, but is reinforced by preparation, delivery and peer evaluation.

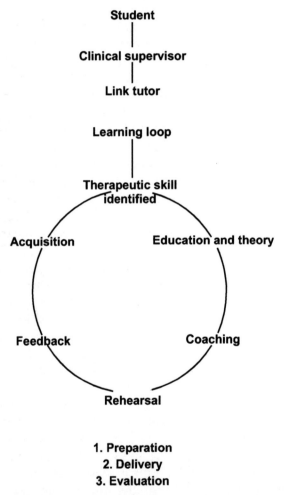

Figure 2.2: Therapeutic Skills Acquisition Model (Morrissey, 2001)

Core skills were identified above, which indicated that many students are not a finished product at the end of their course

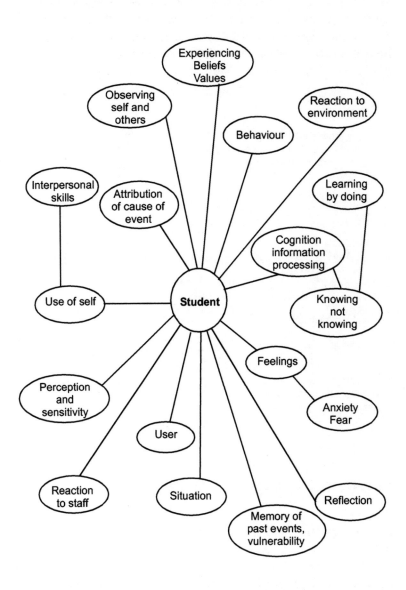

Becoming a mental health nurse

and continue to learn, especially just after qualifying. Perhaps we need to distinguish between surface level competency and deep level competency where the nurse is both confident and competent. However, what is clear is that becoming a mental health nurse is about learning and doing and much more complex than it appears. Mental health nursing is very much

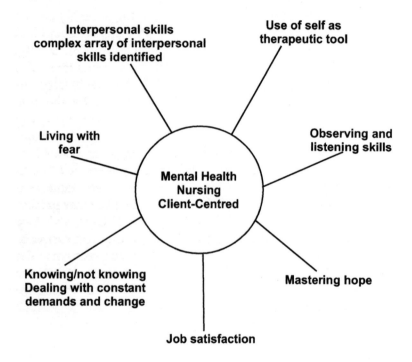

Becoming a mental health nurse: Students' experiences

affected by the conditions of practice and the fact that nurses seem to be expected to deliver wherever there is a need. In reality, it seems that there are many conflicts of interest in the process of becoming a mental health nurse. The above research has proved informative in understanding the lives of student nurses. It has also identified new ways of conceptualising the journey in becoming a mental health nurse. Another important step in future research is to identify ways of bridging the theory practice gap.

Throughout history, nurses have been central to dealing with many forms of mental distress and crisis. To this day, we are still defining our place, our space with users, other mental health professionals, voluntary and statutory organisations and society. We are only visible to those who really need us, and often, we are only valued and respected by those who have been there and come back to tell the tale, namely clients or users. However, more and more nurses spend less and less time involved in therapeutic work (Sullivan, 1998). Surely, investing in students for three years to become mental health nurses is a waste, if they are then unable to engage therapeutically with users. More importantly, who will be the role models for students? If therapeutic relationships are not being formed, surely we are deskilling the nurses we have and depriving users of the care these nurses were trained to deliver. Furthermore, giving a person with a mental health problem a place to live is useless unless there are social networks in place (Blacker and Clare, 1987). Unlike other professionals, nurses see more of the misery and distress, and they cannot leave. They are there for the duration. You can only truly appreciate the work of nurses when you recognise the intensity of their work and their loyalty to users. Whatever may be said about nursing, one person can make a positive and significant contribution to the mental and emotional well being of another human being.

The voice of a user

'I didn't think I'd ever get better, I was so scared and all around me was so strange and chaotic... but Jeremy, the nurse, was so understanding... I still can't believe it happened... I'm sorry I feel so tearful even now... It's silly really but I can remember the admission vividly. I was so incredibly scared but Jeremy was so thoughtful and kind... This gave me some hope... it saved my life... he is really a great nurse ... a really good person. I was lucky I guess.'

The journey in becoming a mental health nurse

References

Altshul A (1972) *Patient-Nurse Interaction: A Study of Interaction Patterns in Acute Psychiatric Wards*. Churchill Livingstone, Edinburgh

Barker P (1999) Common sense caring. *Nurs Stand* 13(44): 22

Blacker C, Clare A (1987) Depressive disorder in primary care. *Br J Psychiatry* 150: 737–51

Brooking J, Ritter S, Thomas B, eds (1992) *A Textbook of Psychiatric and Mental Health Nursing*. Churchill Livingstone, Edinburgh

Burnard P (1991) A method of analysing interview transcripts in qualitative research. *Nurse Educ Today* 11: 461–66

Burnard P (1989) Fads and fashions. *Nurs Times* 85(8): 69–71

Carr P (1979) To describe the role of the psychiatric nurse in a psychiatric unit situated in a district general hospital. PhD thesis. University of Manchester, Manchester

ENB (2002) ENB News: Celebration Highlights from 1983–2002. March: 1–11

Field PA, Morse JM (1994) *Nursing Research: The Application of Qualitative Approaches*. Crohm Helm, London

Gamble C, Brennan G (2001) *Working with Serious Mental Illness: A Manual for Clinical Practice*. Balliere Tindall, Harcourt Publishers Limited, London

Gijbels H (1995) Mental health nursing skills in an acute admission environment: perceptions of mental health nurses and other professionals. *J Adv Nurs* 21(3): 460–65

Glaser B, Strauss A (1967) *The Discovery of Grounded Theory*. Aldine, New York

Gournay K (2000) Suicide and self-harm in in-patient psychiatric units: a study of nursing issues in 31 cases. *J Adv Nurs* 32(1): 124–31

Gournay K (1995) the community psychiatric nurse in primary care: an economic analysis. *J Adv Nurs* 22(4): 769–78

Granskar M, Edberg AK, Fridlund B (2001) Nursing students' experience of their first professional encounter with people having mental disorders. *J Psychiatr Ment Health Nurs* 8: 249–56

50

Hill RG, Hardy P, Shepherd G (1996) *Perspectives on Manic Depression: A Survey of the Manic Depression Fellowship*. The Sainsbury Centre for Mental Health, London

Hammersley M (1992) *What's Wrong with Ethnography?* Routledge, London

Holliday A (2002) *Doing and Writing Qualitative Research*. Sage, London

Morrissey M (2001) Therapeutic skills acquisition model. Cited in: Forster S. *The Role of the Mental Health Nurse*. Stanley Thornes, Cheltenham: Ch 4; 71

Morrissey M (2003) The Journey in Becoming a Mental Health Nurse. APS Publishing, Salisbury - dont think you can do this??

Nolan P (1993) *A History of Mental health Nursing: Theory and Practice*. Chapman and Hall, London

Peplau H (1987) Tomorrow's world. *Nurs Times* 83(1): 29–32

Regel S, Roberts D (2002) *Mental Health Liaison: A Handbook for Nurses and Health Professionals*. Balliere Tindall, Edinburgh

Sainsbury (2002) *Briefing Paper 16: Acute Inpatient Care for People with Mental Health Problems*. Sainsbury Centre for Mental Health, London

Sainsbury (1998) *Briefing Paper 4.: Acute Problems: A Survey of the Quality of Care in Acute Psychiatric Wards*. Sainsbury Centre for Mental Health, London

Sandelowski M (1986) The problem of rigour in qualitative research. *Adv Nurs Sci* 8(3): 27–37

Sullivan P (1998) Therapeutic interaction in mental health nursing. *Nurs Stand* 12(45): 39–42

Watkins P (2001) *Mental Health Nursing; The Art of Compassionate Care*. Butterworth-Heinemann, Oxford

Wilkinson J, Wilkinson C (1996) Group discussions in nursing education: a learning process. *Nurs Stand* 10: 44; 46–47

3

Clinical placements in mental health nursing

'You're not going to ER Ward for your clinical placement, it's terrible there; they say there isn't even one good looking male nurse'.

From the above quote not everyone is looking at their clinical experience in quite the same way.

An important departure from many other university courses is that nurses and mental health nurses are required to do a specific number of clinical placements. These are supervised placements in hospitals and community settings with a variety of client-groups, and are vital to the education of nurses. Students can experience working with or alongside a diversity of health care professionals depending on their placement. In mental health nursing, this presents a number of challenges to students, which need careful consideration. Students can be afraid of being on their own, so a buddy system is a useful option to consider. This encourages support from within a group to offer backup while on placement. This chapter will examine the experiences of students in an assortment of placements and some of the basic preparation and information that needs to be in place. It will also examine ways of improving the variety and quality of placements for future programmes.

Introduction

Popular chat shows, such as Oprah and Kilroy often sensationalise issues surrounding mental health. Such media attention serves the purpose of stereotyping individuals with mental health problems, however unintentional. In reality, it is clear that some of the major health problems today are concerned with mental and emotional health. It is estimated that 1 in 4 of the population will experience a mental health problem at some stage during their life (Klerman, 1987). However, it may be much more prevalent than the figures suggest. Suicide is one of the top ten causes of death in the UK and many of these are young people (Nordencroft *et al*, 2002). Anxiety and depression remain at the top of the list as the most common reason for absence from work in the UK and America (Bower *et al*, 2001; Nolen-Hoeksema, 2001). Alcohol and serious drug problems continue to cost the state in money and lives, for such people are at higher risk of suicide (Nolen-Hoeksema, 2001). A more serious concern is the dramatic rise in childhood consumption of alcohol, ironically, at a time when licensing laws are increasingly relaxed and a policy is in place to make pubs more family friendly (Chapman, 2002) Many people with mental health problems, including the elderly, have diminished, or lack, social support networks and are often lonely and socially disadvantaged (Blacker and Clare, 1987). These people can be desperate for skilled help and social contact.

Of more concern is the growing trend that sees more people with serious mental health problems ending up in prison or on the street. Above all, these individuals need resources, hope and practical support. Historically, voluntary organisations are very much involved with mental health issues. The user movements in the UK are among the strongest in Europe and their co-operative working has achieved substantial improvements for users. Carers' and users' expectations of services has been the focus of much recent psychiatric research (Lelliott *et al*, 2001).

However, it is equality that is at the heart of care for users, and the need for the creation of an enabling culture that promotes human rights, such as the right to work, the right to speak, the right to have pride in oneself, and the right to humane and effective treatment, that is so important. The promotion and protection of human rights for all users must be a standard for care and not just rhetoric. Comfort and protection of a person's dignity is a priority. It is also essential to establish a clear standard for the welfare of nursing staff who sometimes feel guilty for being sick and leaving the ward short of carers.

Mental health nursing is not just about medication management, it is about forging alliances that will help a user to promote and create social networks, to live fulfilling lives and to have fun. Our work as mental health nurses should include facilitating self-help groups (Bower *et al*, 2001) learning and teaching coping skills, social skills (French, 1983), work skills, life skills, relationship skills and survival skills. Mental health nurses are trained in communication and interpersonal skills, and much of their work with users is developmental. If this is not fostered, nurses can become deskilled and task-orientated through no fault of their own. To regain this impetus, there needs to be investment in people, sufficient staffing and skill mix in a suitable friendly and purpose built environment.

In the time in which we now live, it is not unusual for a family to be touched or affected by a serious mental health or emotional problem. There are suggestions that as much as one in every two families are affected (Klerman, 1987). The diversity of care requirements are broad and mental health nursing is an important part of the infrastructure for users.

A placement in a mental health setting could be terrifying for a student nurse who has had little or no experience, either personally or professionally. Many individuals are very sensitive, so it takes care and consideration to prepare students for their first mental health placement. Suggestions will be considered, so that students are in a better position to gain information and support prior to their first experience in mental health. No two students are alike, so careful planning is essential for any placement. It should never be assumed that a student has not had any experience with a mental health problem themselves. For example, a student may have a relative with schizophrenia and even an introductory talk can move them to tears. These issues need to be dealt with sensitively and can help others who may also feel fragile.

It is important that universities offering courses in mental health nursing do not underestimate the anxiety experienced by students concerning their first mental health placement in and outside of the UK (Granskar *et al*, 2001; Morrissey, in press). Furthermore, questions have been levelled at the objectivity involved in assessing nursing practices (O'Neill and McCall, 1996). Yet, the same authors acknowledge that experiential learning allowed a much more adult and independent approach for student learning for practice. Concern has been expressed that certain universities might even abolish mental health and learning disability placements for first year students (Anonymous, 2000). In an Australian study, it is suggested that students can feel more clinically confident, even after one placement (Bell *et al*, 1998). Indeed, positive clinical placements can actually encourage more favourable attitudes to mental health nursing (Martin and Happell, 2001).

In the UK, student concerns have indicated a number of important issues attached to going on their first mental health placement. These will be outlined in more detail later (Morrissey, in press). This may be one area in which lecturer/ practitioners have the potential to make a major contribution, as they often spend a significant amount of time working in practice and at university. This can be a useful resource in finding better and more effective ways of preparing and supporting students in clinical practice.

Another important consideration is having clear guidelines for students in the event of a serious incident or crisis. This is often provided by policies or guidelines in practice placements. This is of utmost importance, given that a single serious incident could cause serious trauma to the student.

If students speak to the manager or visit the placement prior to beginning their care experience, it can have the advantage of reducing the anxiety of the first day. Safety is a priority and it is prudent to provide information about their role, who to contact, how they can be contacted and any questions they may have in any preparation for practice. It is important to understand that we not only prepare students for their first mental health placement, but all placements during their course of study. The next section will explore the experience of a student on her first mental health placement in a work rehabilitation setting.

My first clinical placement in mental health: Diary extracts from a student nurse

Thoughts before

My name is Tessa, I am twenty nine years old, a single parent with two children aged six and eight. We are presently moving house, which is stressful and exciting. I am also in the process of writing my second essay and awaiting the results of my first. I am looking forward to my first placement in mental health, but at the same time I am nervous and worried that I won't fit in and be accepted. I have no idea what to expect.

I'm aware that it is a work rehabilitation centre, but I've never been in one and can only guess that the clients are getting over their illnesses and working to get out into a permanent workplace. I have no idea what mental health problem the clients have and this is also a worry.

Another problem is that I don't drive and so I have to catch a bus and then walk to my placement, which is quite a distance. I have had a telephone conversation with my CPS (clinical practice supervisor), who is also the manager who is called John.

My first day

The manager was not there, which I was made aware of when I spoke on the 'phone. The secretary, Miranda, introduced me to everyone and I had no idea who were staff and who were client's. Andrew, a staff member, showed me the printing machines that are used by staff and clients who were all around a table checking pressure valves. By 11.30 am, I was wondering what the hell I was doing here. What had valves got to do with nursing? Everyone seems really friendly, in fact I can't believe how laid back this place is. I'm also concerned about just how friendly I'm supposed to get with a client. A lot of the clients want to know personal things like where I live and about my family. I am not sure whether I should tell them, as I don't know what they are like. I wish someone at the University had explained all of this. I had been dreading lunchtime, sitting around not knowing who was who and what to say to them.

However, they were great with me. In the afternoon checked valves again; must be the most boring job in the world, but I have learned so much about communicating and I can see just what I am getting from the experience here. I am learning a lot from the people here. I've learned that two people suffer with depression. All in all it's been a good first day but I won't be surprised if I dream about valves in my sleep.

Day 2

Valves again. Met John today; seems friendly and everyone talks highly of him. I couldn't believe what I heard today. A group of clients were sitting around having a friendly discussion about who was nuttier than who. Then they asked me who I thought was the daftest. I just gave a stupid grin. Bernice asked me if I ever got depressed, I nearly choked on my coffee. I'm going to have to ask John how to respond when people ask me such questions. I really didn't know what to say.

Day 3

Today I met Charles, he has got Picks Disease, poor sod; he's only 42 and I can't get over how positive he is. I spent a lot of time chatting to him. They all know who I am, that I am a student nurse and no-one is threatened by this. I was concerned they would be unsure of me, as I am a stranger and may even think I was being nosey. This wasn't so and they seemed eager to talk to me about themselves.

They joked and asked if I really wanted to train to look after idiots like them. I was the only one who didn't laugh. I spoke to John about my fears of saying the wrong thing. I learned about what empathy really means. He was right; they weren't looking for sympathy and didn't want wrapping in cotton wool. They just want to be treated like a 'normal person.' I must learn to see the person first not the illness.

Day 4

Today I went out delivering leaflets in a local town. This gave me a proper chance to speak to some of the others. The people were not clients, but people who are vulnerable to the stresses that most of us would take for granted. It's worrying really and it has made me aware that we all have the potential to be mentally ill. At lunchtime we were discussing about a mother who abused her child and some of the people were getting quite worked up about it.

It's really sad that people diagnosed with mental illness are often assumed to be dangerous. I walked around with Dave as I thought he was staff. He used to be a psychiatric nurse until he had a nervous breakdown after his wife left him. At University it's so easy to forget what it's like to work with many of the issues in practice. I also nearly forgot my next essay is due in next Monday.

Day 5: Final Day

I really enjoyed the placement and the people here were really great to be with. Michael was an absolute darling. He brought me a going away present (a teddy bear) I wanted to cry. He brought in some photos of when he was younger in America. He desperately wants to go back but can't. I had cards from staff and clients and they had hand painted some ornaments and wished me luck for the future. Saying goodbye was not easy. And reflecting on my experience at University, I felt much of the theory was levelled at adult nurses and really not made relevant to mental health nurses at all.

Student concerns

From the above diary it is clear that the student had a number of concerns, before and during her placement, which are echoed by other student experiences. In summary, students might feel anxious and unprepared, need information specifically about mental health, mental disorder, practical information, which includes information concerning transport, the actual placement they are going on and the process of assessment during practice (Morrissey, in press). Students also need realistic learning goals for each placement. More than this, there is a need for good communication between the teacher and the clinical placement, the need to be in touch with the reality of the demands of each clinical placement, including individual concerns of students and CPSs (clinical practice supervisors). Clearly, there are practical issues for effective preparation and liaison between student, tutor, practice supervisor, practice co-ordinators and other relevant staff. The data below shows how students felt before and after a placement (Morrissey, in press). It is clear that lack of preparation of students for placements increases already high levels of anxiety.

Anxiety and support; experience and attitude change

'Felt a bit scared; wondered if every patient was going to be like Hannibal Lector. After placement, I reflected and found it to be a very interesting field of nursing, because I had experienced what it was like to work on a mental health ward. I was pleased to leave ideas about Hannibal Lector in the film where they belong.'

(Female student; 20-year-old)

'I was really anxious about what to expect, and it was difficult what to ask questions about when you have had no experience in this field. I felt I was not really supported well by my clinical supervisor, even though she seemed friendly and helpful. She was always busy and this meant we didn't have much time to talk about things I wanted to learn. My views on mental health changed after this placement. I found my thoughts were much more positive about people with mental health problems'

(Female student; 26-year-old.)

'My clinical supervision was very good. I had a lot of time for group discussion and counselling was offered individually. The groups were open and clients could come and go as they pleased. After this placement, my views of mental health did change. I felt I could now understand more and relate to how some people can't cope with everyday situations and why at some time in their life may need help.'

(Female student; 44-year-old)

'I was anxious before I went on placement. Once on placement it was very enjoyable. I was a bit apprehensive at first, but the whole experience was enjoyable. The staff were friendly. I found it difficult to watch ECT (electro convulsive therapy) and not to let the patients' problems upset me too much. My views of mental *health changed dramatically after the experience on an acute ward. The patients had real problems and they needed support; they were ill and needed treatment. My first views on mental health definitely changed. Mentally ill patients are not all mad!'*

(Female student; 21-year-old)

Many students on placement quickly realise the difference between the world of the university and clinical placements. The main difference is the environment and culture. Some students adapt quite quickly, but others perceive some environments as being oppressive and stressful. Many students describe having to conform to others' standards and beliefs and often feel disempowered and afraid of making mistakes.

'I worry about cocking up, failing; also, strangely, I worry about having to conform to the ways of more established staff—particularly if I believe they are wrong, or I think they are.

(Female student; 45-year-old)

All students need to be introduced to key people in each area of practice and being shy is perhaps one feeling to which many people can relate. In fact, new staff nurses may also experience this when they start in their first post. All acute wards in mental health are not the same. The major difference is not simply the environment, but also how care is organised, managed, the culture, staffing, and the client groups.

Lack of preparation and perception of care

'I didn't know what to expect, whether it was going to be like an institution or more relaxed. It would have been useful to see videos about current placements and issues surrounding mental health nursing.'

(Female student: 23-years-old)

'It would have been useful if a user could have talked to students about their experience. There is a need to provide a lecture before practice on mental health conditions and what our role is and gain real insights into what it's like to have a mental health problem. I have worked for five years already in a mental health setting. I did not enjoy my placement in that the quality of care

given to these people was poor. They had nothing to do all day, but smoke themselves to death and take their medication. I felt their real problems were not addressed and they were offered no real hope for their futures.'

(Female student: 29-years-old)

The above quotes are from real people and indicate that students' anxieties with regard to clinical placements need to be addressed, including concerns about care, university and the support of clinical staff. The next part of the chapter will examine ways of preparing students for mental health placements by providing information, engaging students on a buddy system, identifying the people to communicate with at university and, in practice, providing videos to watch on mental health issues, and a reading list in advance of preparation for practice.

Preparing students for mental health practice

It is important to start by offering a number of introductions based on what students want to know and need to know. It is perhaps impossible to totally prepare students for any clinical placement; however, it is possible to give information, guidance and support. The section will first offer a general introduction, an introduction to mental health, types of mental disorder, and ways of making sure you are prepared for your placement.

Many students are anxious about their placement, particularly if it is their first (Granskar *et al*, 2001; Morrissey, in press). Many students find they are more relaxed when they have contacted their practice supervisor by telephone or even better, arranged to visit the placement before they start, by speaking to the manager of the service. Generally speaking, the services can give you much of the information about the service over the telephone. Some may even e-mail you the information. This gives students a clear mental picture of where they are going. On a more practical note, they will then know how to get there and can be sure of the time involved getting from A to B. When students meet in a group for preparation for practice, this is a good time to talk about creating a buddy system. In essence, this is a system where each member of the group pairs up, and this will be a method of support during the placements. Each group may want to offer support in different ways; for example, a telephone call at work or at home, going on breaks, when possible together, and perhaps meeting as small groups. Distance is a reality and for some a telephone call might be all that is possible. This is just an idea as students sometimes feel lonely or isolated on placement. Once you start your placement, you need to take responsibility for punctuality and agreed meetings. You will need to be familiar with key policies in mental health, for instance, health and safety, and confidentiality. There are other documents with which to become familiar, including the National Service Framework for Mental Health, The Care Programme Approach (CPA), The Mental Health Act, and The Capable Practitioner. There is always an orientation to each service and, usually, you will be introduced to other staff. There should be an agreed learning agenda for each type of student and a discussion about how this can be achieved by the clinical placement. If uncertain, you can always check this out with your clinical supervisor or mentor.

Placements

Placements are often brief and can pose problems for those students who already have a specific interest in, for example, the care of people with eating disorders.

'My clinical work is often quite limited in the sense that you can't really get that involved with a client's care if you are finishing in a couple of weeks. In particular, I don't feel able to develop the skills I would like as you keep moving on. It's hard to explain, apart from saying some of the interaction in nursing is more like being social which is important. But at this stage I am more interested in developing communication skills, and learning about interventions to change behaviour.'

(Student; Year 3)

Unlike clinical psychology trainees or medical students, nursing placements are weeks not months. It is only at the end of the course that students get the chance to work for longer periods, often when essays and assessments are already complete or nearing completion. Initially, students need to orientate themselves to the placement and the staff they are working with. In particular, it is important to have an understanding of what the service is and what it offers to users and others. As mentioned in an earlier chapter about becoming a mental health nurse, students often feel as if they are always the new boy or girl.

You may genuinely feel that you are always introducing yourself to someone new, and this can be stressful. Some students also mentioned how important it was for them to be liked. In reality, you cannot be liked by everyone and so, from an early stage, it is important to equip yourself with that basic fact. If there are problems on the placement, it is important to discuss them early with your mentor. It is important to deal with such problems early, so that issues can be dealt with promptly. Potentially, many problems can arise in practice, yet the majority can be sorted out very informally and efficiently. The manager is another resource person and your personal tutor if for any reason there is a problem with talking to your mentor or CPS.

Introduction to mental health

Many students want a textbook description of mental health. There are many available and these often offer a Western medical perspective rather than a holistic nursing perspective. More than this, many definitions are ethnocentric and do not always look at the global and transcultural picture of mental health (Fernando, 2002). However, it is useful to give factual information, general definitions and working definitions about mental health, the various types of mental disorders and common treatment methods. Equally, students want to know what the role of a nurse is and the role of other allied professionals. They also want to know the type of placements available and the client groups they are likely to encounter. This section will offer a brief description of mental health focussing on these points, emphasising the knowledge and skills of mental health nurse.

Definitions

Defining health or mental health is far from straight forward and it seems the more they are defined the more elusive their everyday meaning becomes. The World Health Report (WHO, 2000: xi) defines the objective of good health as two-fold: 'the best attainable average level-goodness-and the smallest feasible difference among individuals and groups-fairness'. However, this definition has not been without criticism and some authors claim it is full of paradoxes when you look at health as a global phenomenon (Fernando, 2002).

Of more concern is the fact that it is not clear what is meant by mental health in a world context. Perhaps there is a need to define mental health in different ways. For example, if you are going to use mental health as a defining or umbrella term about oppression of minorities (Fernando, 2002), can you use mental health in the same way in relation to understanding depression? Can you talk about certain cultural practices that are inhumane as an illness? Another interesting view suggests that mental health is 'the aftertaste of a society's other activities, the residue of all its policies.' (Karpf, 1988). What is clear is that the concept of mental health is very different when considered cross-culturally (Fernando, 2002; White, 1982). For the purposes of this section, it is necessary to provide some working definitions of mental health and mental disorder, types of mental disorder and to outline some common treatments.

Working definitions

'The ability to deal with the recurrent stresses of living and make a relatively effective adjustment.'

(Thomas et al, 1997)

'A dynamic state in which thought, feeling, and behaviour that is age appropriate and congruent with the local and cultural norms is demonstrated.'

(Thomas et al, 1997)

'Maladaptive responses to stressors from the internal or external environment, evidenced by thoughts, feelings, and behaviours that are incongruent with the local and cultural norms, and interfere with the individuals social, occupational, and/or physical functioning.'

(Townsend, 1996)

All the above definitions try to define mental health. However, none of them mention spiritual health, emotional health, or view mental health holistically. Clearly, the environment and the person need to be considered in any definition. In everyday language, a person has a mental health problem when:

'Their life is out of their normal balance, they are no longer able to perform, need assistance or have great difficulty performing normal everyday tasks; they are suffering emotionally and psychologically and the quality of life, including their social relations, is severely affected. In some cases, their partner and friends may be the only ones to notice bizarre behaviour which is out of their normal repertoire.'

(Morrissey, in press).

The diagnosis of common mental health problems or mental disorder can be complex and problematic. In the UK, assessments can be done in people's own homes and in hospital, usually by a psychiatrist. However, mental health nurses and social workers are increasingly involved in assisting and doing assessments. Anxiety and depression remain the most common mental health problem today (Nolen-Hoeksema, 2001). Frequently, general practitioners may lack training in mental health, and diagnosis for some people can take years (Hill *et al*, 1996). Ninety percent of mental health problems are dealt with in primary care (Goldburg, 1995), yet many people will not get the help they need until they have relapsed. Many people with acute mental health problems are unlikely to attend a general practitioner without assistance and many suffer the stigma of being mentally ill. Of more concern is the growing pressure on acute services, which are often under-resourced and understaffed (Sainsbury, 1998). Students often ask for a basic outline of the types of mental disorder. The list below is only a few of the many types of mental disorder defined; it does, however, list the most commonly occurring mental disorders:

- alcohol and drug dependance
- anxiety and depression
- mood disorders
- bi-polar disorder, post natal depression
- childhood disorders e.g autism, depression
- obsessive compulsive disorder
- psychosis e.g. schizophrenia, puerpural psychosis, drug induced psychosis
- eating disorders, anorexia nervosa/bulimia
- behavioural disorders
- personality disorders
- dementia.

The two major systems for categorisation and diagnosis of mental disorder are ICD10 (WHO, 1992), which refers to the International Classification System and DSM (American Psychiatric Association, 1994) refers to the Diagnostic Statistical Manual.

The main treatments for mental disorder fall into a number of categories: chemotherapy or medication, therapeutic, psychological (including psychotherapy), counselling, behavioural, and nursing interventions. The main types of care for depression are initially an assessment then a diagnosis, if one is possible, which usually includes a period of observation. If the depression is defined as a reactive depression, then it needs to be decided if it is best treated psychologically; for example, using counselling or some other method. The rates of mental health problems vary, but some researchers have offered a guide (Strathedee *et al*, 1997). Students need to read around the subject and references that may be of interest are included at the end of this chapter (Gamble and Brennan, 2000; Regel and Roberts 2002; Stuart and Sundeen, 1997; Watkins, 2001).

Mental health disorders (Strathedee *et al*, 1997)

Diagnosis	Rates per 1000 Population per year	Number of patients per year in a practice of 1900
Schizophrenia	2–6	4–12
Active psychosis	3.0	6–7
Organic dementia	2.2	4–5
Depression	30–50	60–100
Anxiety and other neuroses	35.7	70–80
Situational disturbances/other diagnoses	26.7	50–60
Drug and Alcohol dependency	2.7	5–6
Personality disorder (severe)	1.1	2–3

First clinical placement

In your first placement you are not expected to know about mental health in any depth and most clinicians will be expecting to teach you the basics. This includes helping to settle you into your first placement. The role of the student in practice is to be clear about your learning objectives, your clinical supervisor and mentor. You also need to gain practical knowledge about the placement you are going on and learn to take responsibility for yourself, which is a longer term aspect of learning. If you are unsure of anything, i.e. taking a blood pressure, you are free to ask for assistance. Equally, if you would like to sit in on a meeting—say with a clinical psychologist—this too is encouraged. Your first placement is always an anxious time for students unless you have had experience before in this area.

Discussion

The above section outlines some very basic facts about mental health, and it becomes clear that students need to be prepared for placement and have time to discuss any anxieties or fears. Written information alone will not necessarily reassure students, so there needs to be preparation sessions prior to each placement. It is also good practice to have an evaluation of each placement, so that any clinical or learning difficulties can be identified. It is evident that students can gain more out of a placement if they are adequately prepared. Increasingly, students are involved in finding their own placements in specialist areas. However, these need to be vetted appropriately.

References

American Psychiatric Association (1994) *Diagnostic and Statistical Manual of Mental Disorders*, 4th edn. (DSM VI) American Psychiatric Association, Washington, DC

Bell A, Horsfall J, Goodwin W (1998) The mental health nursing clinical confidence scale: a tool for measuring undergraduate learning on mental health clinical placements. *Aus N Z J Ment Health Nurs* 7: 184–90

Blacker C, Clare A (1987) Depressive disorder in primary care. *Br J Psychiatry* 150: 737–51

Bower P, Richards D, Lovell K (2001) The clinical effectiveness of self-help treatments for anxiety and depressive disorders in primary care: a systematic review. *Br J Clin Pract* 51(471): 838–45

Chapman J (2002) Childhood drinking doubles in a decade. *Daily Mail* Tuesday November 5: 16

Fernando S (2002) *Mental Health Race and Culture*, 2nd edn. Palgrave, Hampshire

French P (1983) *Social Skills for Nurses*. Croom Helm, Kent

Gamble C, Brennan G (2000) *Working with Serious Mental Illness. A Manual for Clinical Practice*. Bailliere Tindall, London

Goldburg D (1995) The Fields Trials of the Mental Disorders Section of ICD-10 designed for primary care in England. *Fam Pract* **12**(4)

Granskar M, Edberg AK, Fridlund B (2001) Nursing students' experience of their first professional encounter with people having mental disorders. *J Psychiatr Ment Health Nurs* **8**: 249–56

Hill RG, Hardy P, Shepherd G (1996) *Perspectives on Manic Depression: A Survey of the Manic Depression Fellowship.* The Sainsbury Centre for Mental Health, London

Karpf A (1988) ' Why We Get Bad Health by Media', *The Guardian*, 11: May 21

Klerman GL (1987) Psychiatric epidemiology and mental health policy. In: Levine S, Lilienfield A, eds. *Epidemiology and Health Policy.* Tavistock, New York: 227–64

Lelliott P, Beevor A, Hogman G, Hyslop J, Lathlean J, Ward M (2001) Carers' and users' expectations of services-user version (CUES-U): a new instrument to measure mental health services. *Br J Psychiatry* **179**: 67–72

Martin T, Happell B (2001) Undergraduate nursing students' views of mental health nursing in the forensic environment. *Aus N Z J Ment Health Nurs* **10**(2): 116–25

Morrissey M (in press) Becoming a mental health nurse the experience: a qualitative study. *Int J Psychiatr Nurs Res*

Nolen-Hoeksema S (2001) *Abnormal Psychology,* 2nd edn. McGraw Hill, Boston

Nordencroft M, Jeppersen P, Abel M, *et al* (2002) OPUS study: suicidal behaviour, suicidal ideation, and hopelessness among patients with first episode psychosis: One-year follow up of a randomised controlled trial. *Br J Psychiatry* **181**(43): S98–S106

O'Neill A, McCall J ((1996) Objectively assessing nursing practices: a curricular development. *Nurse Educ Today* **16**: 121–26

Regel S, Roberts D (2002) *Mental Health Liaison: A Handbook for Nurses and Health Professionals.* Balliere Tindall, Edinburgh

Sainsbury Centre for Mental Health (1998) *Briefing Paper 4: Acute Problems: A Survey of the Quality of Care in Acute Psychiatric Wards.* Sainsbury Centre for Mental Health, London

Strathedee G, Kendrick T, Cohen A, Thompson K (1997) *A General Practitioner's Guide to Managing Long Term Mental Health Disorders*. The Sainsbury Centre for Mental Health, London

Stuart GW, Sundeen SJ eds (1997) *Mental Health Nursing Principals and Practice*, UK edn. Mosby, London

Thomas B, Hardy B, Cutting P (1997) In: Stuart GW, Sundeen SJ, eds. *Mental Health Nursing: Principles and Practice*, UK edn. Mosby, London

Townsend CR (1996) *Ecology: Individuals, Populations and Communities*. Blackwell Scientific, Oxford

Watkins P (2001) *Mental Health Nursing; The Art of Compassionate Care*. Butterworth-Heinemann, Oxford

White GM (1982) Ethnographic study of cultural knowledge of mental disorder. In: Marsella AJ, White GM, eds. *Cultural Concepts of Mental Health and Therapy*. Reidel, Dordrecht: 69–95

WHO (2000) *Guide to Mental Health in Primary Care*. Royal Society of Medicines Press, London

WHO (1992) *ICD-10: Classification of Mental and Behavioural Disorders*. World Health Organization, Geneva

Further reading

Aggleton P, Hurry J (2000) *Young People and Mental Health*. John Wiley & Son, Chichester

Barris R (1998) *Bodies of Knowledge in Psychosocial Practice*. Blackwell Scientific, Oxford

Castillo RJ (1998) *Meanings of Madness*. Brooks/Cole Publishing Company, Thompson Corporation, London

Forster S (2001) *The Role of the Mental Health Nurse*. Stanley-Thornes, Gloucester

Gamble C, Brennan G (2000) *Working with Serious Mental Illness: A Manual for Clinical Practice*. Bailliere Tindall, London

Reynolds A, Thornicroft G (1999) *Managing Mental Health Services*. Open University Press, Buckingham

The Maudsley NHS Trust (1997) The Maze Mental Health Act 1983 Guidelines. The Maudsley NHS Trust, London

4

Creating a learning atmosphere using group work and experiential learning

Each day you may be surrounded by people in a busy social world, yet feel isolated, lonely, and unconnected. In the egocentric culture in which we live, many people feel alienated and have little experience of being valued as part of a group, a community or society. In today's consumer culture, there is a lack of motivation towards being interested in you, unless there is something tangible in it for them. If living in such a society presents difficulties for an ordinary person, it is hard to imagine the barriers faced by a person with a serious mental health disorder. Being part of a group can initiate powerful connections in learning and social communication, which can then be used to help others. More importantly, this can help students to learn about the importance of valuing themselves; their social networks, coping, social, and living skills, and therapeutic communication skills. Only when you sit with users of mental health services can you start to appreciate the challenge and value in developing and providing groups and group work skills in mental health. Group work can foster hope, social networks, and is a place where people can be valued as individuals and not as an illness or as a victim. Understanding of group processes can be informative and useful in learning about ourselves, as many authors testify (Brown, 2000; Doughlas, 1995; Durkin, 1995).

> 'I enjoy coming to the group here at the day hospital; it's good to see people and you don't feel so useless; we encourage each other and the atmosphere is nice. We share a joke sometimes.'
>
> (User)

'To be honest I don't have any real motivation, but I enjoy this group as it gives me a feeling that it is worth trying. Sometimes it's hard because of the voices, but it is nice having other people around and I miss that when I go back to my flat.'

(User)

'I guess you lose so much at the start. I mean you don't want a mental illness, I am still fighting that I guess, but then there is so much prejudice to contend with. People say it must be awful but they really don't know the half of it. It's hard for me when I see my friends, wishing it was me. When I have a relapse, I sometimes go to hospital and I am with much older people who are often very disturbed; it feels so desperate, alien, the place people and experiences. I'm 23 years old and I am not stupid, but I know I have schizophrenia. People are so ignorant; you can see the way they respond. When I'm well I take the medication but, when I'm not, it gets overtaken by the voices. I certainly wouldn't put schizophrenia down on my CV. It is really frightening, truly a living hell and soon after recovery, it starts again; the fear of relapse, trying to keep things together, contending with hallucinations.'

(User)

There needs to be more groups for individuals, partners and families of people with mental health problems, as illustrated by one husband about his wife who has bipolar mood disorder. In this disorder the person experiences severe mood fluctuations at times, known as highs, where the person becomes elated, hyperactive, disinhibited, and can loose touch with reality. The lows are indicated by mild to clinical depression. Contrary to many beliefs, these symptoms can go undetected by the person and others around them. What is needed is family education, support and group work for individuals and partners.

'When my wife is depressed, it obviously has an enormous effect on my life; my confidence is definitely reduced because I feel so inadequate, I'd go off the chart. When she feels good I feel very positive.'

(Hill *et al*, 1996)

Given the serious and personally challenging nature of much of the work of student nurses, learning in a group provides a safe space and can develop confidence. This chapter will focus on some exciting and fun ways for students to learn about people skills in mental health nursing, using experiential learning and group work. The classroom needs to be exciting for students to learn (Bonwell and Eison, 1991) and so, too, does the need to create a learning atmosphere . While lectures are the norm in universities as a teaching method, they are not the only method and might be very limited in relation to the acquisition of skills and knowledge for mental health nursing.

Nursing departments need to facilitate the use of group work and experiential learning, if they want to generate real learning and critical thinking for nursing practice. This is evidenced by much research (Jaques, 2000; Lauder 1996; McAllister, 1996; Race, 2000; Wallace, 1996; Wilkinson and Wilkinson, 1996). Yet, it seems such methods of learning are often not employed in many nursing departments, and are frequently viewed less favourably than traditional teaching methods. Users of mental health services need social and therapeutic groups (Hill *et al*, 1996).

Small groups put students at the centre of learning. The concept of a 'small group' is not simply defined by the number of students involved, it is the purpose that defines it. It gives students a chance to exchange ideas, experience face to face contact, mirror clinical practice experiences. Numbers greater than 20 impede the outcomes of learning. Group work involves exploring concepts, such as social roles, group norms, boundaries, conformity and decision, etc. A climate of acceptance, support, and trust needs to be fostered (Quinn, 1995). Group skills and group work are essential for those becoming mental health nurses. In the future, departments should be given resources to establish rooms specially designed for the purpose of developing the skills of mental health nursing students.

Frequently, resources are available in universities to provide skills laboratories for adult nursing. Similar resources should be available for mental health nurses. Such rooms should provide soft chairs, in a comfortable, well ventilated, light room. A method for recording groups and interviews for teaching and research purposes would also be useful.

The greatest benefits of group work and experiential learning are increased personal and professional development (Hartley, 1997; Tiberius, 1999). It provides a safe place for people to be themselves, and has the advantage of encouraging weaker members of the group, facilitating change, thought to be impossible by some students. Furthermore, although not written into the nursing curriculum, students need to know they have learned a new skill and they need feedback from their practice.

If they fail to receive such feedback, students can lack confidence, even with what they do know. As part of this group process, students can be given useful feedback by members of their own group. This is useful in relation to their performance on group tasks, in role play, or in learning practical and communication skills with other group members. It is also a useful gauge with which students can monitor their learning and general performance, given that all the students are focussed on the same qualification, especially during branch programmes in mental health nursing. Specifically, group work remains an important tool in learning interpersonal skills.

Such skills are important, if we are to reach people diagnosed with cancer, for example, who can suffer depression, often without communicating their suffering (Ogden, 2000). Group work provides a platform to learn interview skills, how to develop confidence and assertiveness, improve self-esteem, cope with difficult feelings, deal with fear and rejection, counselling skills, etc. From this comes the development of advanced skills and knowledge, using group work to prepare mental health nursing students for practice. Teachers should offer advance preparation for these sessions, so that students can prepare themselves, and students need to be supportive of the teacher in creating a 'learning atmosphere'. Initially, some individuals find group work difficult, but these are often the ones who gain most from the sessions.

Group work

Few people could learn a skill, particularly a complex one, by lecture notes alone, thus there is a need to look more closely at how student nurses learn and how to make their learning more effective and more enjoyable.

What is group work? The answer depends to some extent on the person you ask. In essence, the setting in which workers practice determines many of the differences. There is a different focus to groups; groups with a personal orientation, interpersonal groups, and groups addressing social concerns. In turn, the influence of the workplace on practice is not a matter of chance, and group work is offered in many different settings, from hospitals to training institutions (Manor, 2000).

Development and growth through group work can be painful. Despite the purpose of groups being to help us to learn more about ourselves, try out new behaviours and improve the way we communicate, we often resist this process because it is demanding, requires energy and is frightening. Dynamics in groups mean that individual members feel under pressure to engage in self-disclosure, intimacy and confrontation. The consequence is to make us re-evaluate our perceptions of ourselves—our conceptual framework—and can precipitate anxiety, shame, guilt and other uncomfortable feelings. There is a natural tendency to avoid such feelings. Avoidance behaviour or defensive behaviours are ingrained and unconscious.

Defence mechanisms in groups

As such defences interfere with personal and group development, it is vital to recognise and deal with them effectively. Generally, all defences are evasive in nature; such manoeuvres may be categorised by whether the individual moves toward (fight) or away from (flight) the source of conflict or chooses to manipulate other group members (pairing). For the purposes of this text, a basic outline will be given as an introduction (Thoresen, 1972).

Fight defenses

These are based on the premise that 'the best defence is a good offence.'

Competition with the facilitator: The person who struggles to control the group or 'outdo' the trainer may be attempting to prove his/her group prowess in order to avoid dealing with his/her own behaviour.

Cynicism: This is manifested by frequent challenging of the group contract and goals, sceptical questioning of genuine behaviour, and attacks on stronger, threatening members.

Interrogation: A barrage of proving questions keeps others in the group on the defensive. An individual who habitually cross-examines others under the guise of 'gaining helpful information and under-standing' may be fighting to keep the spotlight safely away from her-self.

Group work means being part of a group or it can mean being a facilitator, and each student needs to learn how to do this in order to run groups themselves. To be in a group can provide experiences that students take with them into practice, and also helps to gain a feeling for the support and interaction of fellow students. Students are given the opportunity to question, to understand, to discuss issues and, later, to challenge and confront. There are many types of groups; open, closed, encounter groups, therapeutic groups (Egan, 1976), and groups in hospitals, churches, schools, etc. For simplicity, Tuckman (1965) put forward five stages of group development.

Tuckman (1965) The sequences of group development

Forming	coming together Getting started	
Storming	honeymoon over Interpersonal conflicts Rivalry over power/structure 'fight', 'flight'	**Phase 1 Power Relationships**
Norming	getting down to it Working relationships established Atmosphere clearer Issues dealt with Process and task separated	

****

Performing	getting on with it Planning targets met or revised Relationships not a preoccupation Satisfaction in achievements	**Phase 2 Personal Relationships**
Mourning	closure, loss, flight behaviour by some Minimising achievements Romanticising the past Looking ahead, commitment declines	

Often, students joining a mental health group for the first time start by saying , 'You are not going to make us do role-play, are you?' This can be to do with fear and also to let the teacher know that they have heard from other students about role-play. It is a way of expressing dominance saying, Well, we're not going to be taking any of that, thank you. The fear is to do with performance anxiety; fear of looking stupid, fear of being embarrassed, fear of being forced into the spotlight, to be the focus of unwanted attention.

When the group is new, such activities seem very risky but, as the individuals move through the stages of group development, even in tasks originally seen as scary, they perform well.

'I must admit at the start I really was scared the teacher was going to ask me to join in or ask me a question, a bit like at school. But later on, after I trusted and knew people more, I didn't find role play a problem in fact it was more interesting.'

(Student)

'To be honest I still find groups difficult, I feel more self-conscious, I prefer to be in the background. Since Amy, my friend, has started to speak more in the group, it makes me feel like talking more, it's a gradual thing.'

(Student)

Role play involves acting out a particular scene. For example, asking a person out on a date. The skills for this exercise relate to developing confidence and identifying effective communication skills. Each student is given a script to read and then they decide who is going to be which character in the scene. The facilitator ensures all questions are considered relating to the performance and resources are organised in advance. As is usual, in all managed role plays, students are debriefed and there is a discussion of what they have learned from the experiences. If the role play is planned in advance and students are given a chance to experiment themselves, it can mean they feel less threatened. Students often find it difficult if a role play is suddenly sprung on them and perhaps this is why some students feel so anxious about taking part.

If you have been a member of a group of any kind, you can appreciate many of the issues discussed in this chapter, but if you have never taken part in group work, you will share the concerns of the students. Fears are often concerned with talking in a group, disclosing in a group, being shy or embarrassed, and working with group members who are strangers. Students fear self-disclosure, sitting in a circle feeling vulnerable and self-conscious, worrying about what people think of them, fearing to speak too much, or not being able to speak at all.

A learning atmosphere should be a place that is nurturing, safe and fun, and its value needs to shared by teacher and students together (Morrissey, in press). Creating a learning atmosphere requires people to put effort into the disposition of the physical environment to ensure seating is arranged in a circle, that there is enough natural sunlight, the chairs are comfortable and there are enough learning and teaching resources, etc. Sessions should be planned in advance so that students and the teacher can spend most of their time learning and not going over notes, then the actual learning experience can be the focus and students can be the centre of learning. Once a good rapport is developed between students and teacher, based on respect and flexibility, real adult learning can take place.

> 'The first time I sat in a mental health group as part of my training, I felt naked in a way that I haven't felt before. Introducing myself to other students and being self-conscious of my shaky voice and my body language. However, it broke down some barriers and made me feel I had a place in the crowd.'
>
> (Student)

> 'It made me aware we were different to other students who sat behind desks... don't get me wrong I really was attached to mine... [laugh]. Well setting ground rules was fun... and we were such a big group, twenty two... sometimes we didn't listen to each other one at a time as we were supposed to.... I learned being in a group was not all about keeping to rules and boundaries...it was sometimes challenging these.'
>
> (Student)

The social world in which we live is often busy, diverse and confusing and it is not always easy to understand everyday experiences. There are many demands and more people are realising that they need to develop new skills to survive, cope, communicate and grow as a person. In our social worlds, we spend much of our time checking out our experiences with others from a very early age. One interesting basic observation on human perception is to find that no two people experience the same stimulus in the same way. Perhaps you've had the experience of telling a good joke, and one person laughs hysterically while the other says 'so what!' As individuals, we are unique, just like our sense of humour. Friendship helps us to see the world in new ways and grow and develop as individuals. Learning from experience and being part of group work enables us to express ourselves openly, develop trust and work with fear. It can be a refreshing and engaging way to work with students, users and their families. Given the importance placed on the development of interpersonal skills in the majority of nursing and research texts (Altschul 1972; Gamble and Brennan 2001; Watkins, 2001), it is vital that students are afforded an opportunity to learn and experience group work at first hand. How else can they become competent to take part and develop group work for users in clinical practice?

Experiential learning

Experiential learning is defined in different ways (Wallace, 1996) but, in essence, it is:

> *'Experience followed by reflection, discussion, analysis and evaluation and leads to insight, discovery and understanding, which is then conceptualised, synthesised and integrated into the individual's system of constructs which he/she imposes on the world.'*

(Wight, in Boydell, 1976)

or a more simplified definition:

> *'Experiential learning occurs when a person engages in some activity, looks back at the activity critically, abstracts some useful insight from the analysis and puts the result to work'*
>
> (Heron, 1989; Miles, 1987; Pfieffer and Jones, 1980; Wallace, 1996)

Experiencing your world

Experiencing your world means collecting information and trying to making sense of it. Decision-making, reasoning and prioritising are all important skills to develop for clinical practice. This is important as students spend time in many complex situations personal and professional, in university and in practice. Such learning opportunities are not always valued or used (Fretwell, 1982; Miles, 1987). This is particularly important in relation to learning from practice which needs to be invested in and developed. In the classroom, real life situations are important as are informative case studies, 'Following the Experiential Learning Cycle' (Boydell, 1976; Jones, 1981).

An integral component of experiential learning is reflection on practice (Kolb, 1984 'The Experiential Learning Cycle'). Experiential learning is a very good vehicle for creating critical thinking in the student nurse. This is important as students are required to demonstrate skills of critical analysis in both their academic and clinical work (Schank, 1990). More importantly for mental health nurses, learning new problem-solving skills is essential to their work. Critical thinking can be taught using experiential learning. Critical thinking is a logical process constructed from discrete constituents and a skill that can be taught and learned (Fisher, 1995), although others have disputed this (McPeck, 1990). On balance, it is clear from practice that people can learn new ways of thinking from all kinds of experience. As a mental health nurse, one can learn new ways of thinking and much of this is learned while in practice. Problem-solving in mental health is a skill that is born from labour that can be emotionally and mentally intensive. An interesting method for understanding problem-solving in mental health nursing was recently put forward (Lemmer, 2002).

The Cognitive Sketch Pad ties in well with the earlier model of becoming a mental health nurse where students develop a picture of themselves as practitioners, often through coping with uncertainty in a plethora of experiences. Using the sketch pad echoes previous ideas and theories concerned with cognitive mapping. This helps to explain how conversations with users can be used as data and learning material. Lemmer puts forward a useful way of conceptualising learning and practice using a cognitive sketchpad. What is useful here is that the dialogue of the user is mapped and utilised as data, and the model is developmental and applied to practice. A thought record or mind map is generated, which can create a picture of a user's thoughts, feelings, and behaviours. Such a map can be updated and a much richer data set can be generated, which can be used in therapeutic work.

'In my observation there is a change of mood and attitude in staff and patients during the process of using the Cognitive Sketch Pad to map thoughts, feelings and behaviours' (Lemmer, 2002). As part of the demonstrations to this cognitive approach to care, an introductory briefing is given. This includes written information with an example of the approach in practice. The benefit of such an approach is that it strengthens interaction between nurses and users, creates a structure for interaction and therapy, and offers measurement to the process. The main weakness is perhaps in the amount of data created, its interpretation, the perception of the nurse about how to use this model, and the need to test the method for reliability and validity.

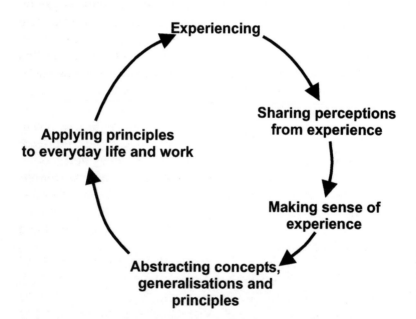

From Boydell (1976 and Pfieffer and Jones 1979

Experimental Learning Cycle

Sharing perceptions from experience

Individuals who have participated in the experience share with others what they saw/or felt during the activity. This makes available to the group the experience of each individual and serves to deepen and broaden perception.

Making sense of the experience

This is the key step in the experiential learning cycle in which individuals make a systematic examination of the common experience. By asking the questions: What did it mean; Is there anything happening here that we all interpret; individuals and the group are able to clarify the meaning of the experience and to begin realising how the information generated by the activity might be used in future experiences.

Abstracting concepts, generalisation and principles

The learners should ask how the concepts, generalisations and principles, abstracted in previous analysis, can be applied in the future. The process could be enhanced by the use of individual goal setting, developmental action plans, and learning contracts. Boydell claims that by using this approach to learning, individuals will achieve 'meta-goals' and abilities that are life pervasive:

> 'To identify and use the resources in a situation; identify, cope with, and turn to advantage the constraints in a situation; obtain co-operation from colleagues in solving problems; cope with uncertainty, ambiguity and the fact that there is no right answer; restructure one's experience and hence learn from it; be sensitive to one's feelings in a situation and to the effect that these are having on one's behaviour.'

(Boydell, 1976)

In light of these developments, it seems that all nurses will need such abilities in the future, including the ability to analyse and report on incidents using frameworks, such as, Critical Incident Analysis (Miles, 1987). The sentiments are echoed more recently (Fisher, 1995; Schank, 1990; Wallace, 1996). Students can only benefit from becoming more conversant with data surrounding incidents in practice. The use of a real case study provides useful discussions for student and teacher. In such a situation, experiential learning brings out critical and evaluative skills in students. Such a method also teaches students how to record aspects of their clinical observations (Gordon and Benner, 1984) and development of critical thinking (Kintgen-Andrews, 1988). A more direct approach is to involve users in the teaching of mental health nursing and, in so doing, inform and challenge the perceptions of students on some of the basic issues to do with care. Having users in an experiential learning programme improves and fosters, at an early stage, a positive and constructive partnership based on real lived experiences. This is useful before students go on their first mental health placement and affirms the users' place in the education of student nurses.

Experiential learning is concerned with learning about facts and processes. The facts are important, but the processes are vital to providing care, which is bound, in part, in the experiences of users and clinicians. One experience can inform the other. As mental health nurses, we need to learn to realise ourselves and the benefits of group and experiential learning. Medication management is only one aspect of being a mental health nurse, but our knowledge and professional abilities can go far beyond that. Group work and experiential learning have given us tools for humanity, respect, dignity, empowerment, compassion, problem-solving, critical thinking, therapeutic skills and interventions, teamwork, assertiveness, interpersonal skills, analysis, new research techniques, social support, social networks, encouragement, reassurance, and hope. Experiential learning forms part of the repertoire of nurse educators and many pre and post-registration curriculum documents focus on the development of the autonomous practitioner, who is able to think critically (Wallace, 1996). Group work and experiential learning need to be valued in education and practice not just for students, but also for the skills they generate. This will be the fabric and vehicle to provide support and dialogue with user needs. Users need more than medication management, they need support and groups. This often provides their only social network (Blacker and Clare, 1987). Without a group to attend, some individuals would be completely alone. Medication will never conquer loneliness, but groups can be a place to be and should be a right for all users.

References

Altschul A (1972) *Patient-Nurse Interaction: A Study of Interaction Patterns in Acute Psychiatric Wards*. Churchill Livingstone, Edinburgh

Blacker C, Clare A (1987) Depressive disorder in primary care. *Br J Psychiatry* **150**: 737–51

Bonwell C, Eison J (1991) *Active Learning/Creating Excitement in the Classroom*. ASHE-ERIC Higher Education, Report No. 1, Washington

Boydell T (1976) *Experiential Learning*. Manchester Monographs No. 5. University of Manchester, Department of Adult Education, Manchester

Brown R (2000) *Group Processes*, 2nd edn. Blackwell Publishers, Oxford

Doughlas T (1995) *Developmental Social Psychology*. Blackwell Publishers, Oxford

Durkin K (1995) *Survival in Groups—The Basics of Group Membership*. Open University Press, Buckinghamshire

Egan G (1976) Confrontation. *Group Org Stud* **1**(2): 223–43

Fisher A (1995) *Infusing Critical Thinking into the College Curriculum*. Centre for Research in Critical Thinking, University of East Anglia, Norwich

Fretwell JE (1982) *Ward Teaching and Learning*. Royal College of Nursing, London

Gamble C, Brennan G (2001) *Working with Serious Mental Illness: A Manual for Clinical Practice*. Balliere Tindall, Harcourt Publishers, London

Gordon DR, Benner P (1984) Guidelines for recording critical incidents, developed by Gordon and Benner. In: Benner P, ed. *From Novice to Expert: Excellence and Power in Clinical*

Nursing Practice. Addison-Wesley Publishing, Menlo Park, CA,

Hartley P (1997) *Group Communication*. Routledge, London

Heron J (1989) *The Facilitators Handbook*. Kogan Page, London

Hill RG, Hardy P, Shepherd G (1996) *Perspectives on Manic Depression; A Survey of the Manic Depression Fellowship*. The Sainsbury Centre for Mental Health, London

Jaques D (2000) *Learning in Groups*, 3rd edn. Kogan Page, London

Jones WJ (1981) Self-directed learning and student-selected goals in nurse education. *J Adv Nurs* 6(1): 59–69

Kintgen-Andrews J (1988) *Development of Critical Thinking: Career Ladder PN and AD Nursing Students, Pre-Health Science Freshmen, Generic Baccalaureate Sophomore Nursing Students*. ERIC ED 297153. Minnesota School of Nursing

Kolb DA (1984) *Experiential Learning*. Prentice Hall, New Jersey; NY

Lauder W (1996) Constructing meaning in the learning experience: the role of alternative theoretical frameworks. *J Adv Nurs* 24: 91–97

Lemmer B (2002) *Cognitive Sketch Pad: Terms for Engagement in the Care of People with Serious Mental Impairment*. Canterbury Christ Church University College, Canterbury

McAllister M (1996) Learning contracts: an Australian experience. *Nurse Educ* 16: 199–205

McPeck JE (1990) *Teaching Critical Thinking, Dialogue and Dialectic*. Routledge and Chapman Hall, New York; NY

Manor O (2000) *Ripples: Groupwork in Different Settings*. Whiting and Birch, London

Miles RJ (1987) Experiential learning in the curriculum: Cited in: Allan P, Moya J. *The Curriculum in Nursing Education*. Croom Helm, London

Morrissey M (in press) The Experience of Becoming a Mental Health Nurse: A qualitative study. *Int J Psychiatr Nurs Res*

Morrissey M (in press) Setting up a learning atmosphere. A student evaluation of learning.*Int J Psychiatr Nurs Res*

Ogden J (2000) *Health Psychology*, 2nd edn. Open University Press, Buckingham

Pfieffer JW, Jones JE (1980) *Structured Experience Kit. Users Guide*, University Associates, San Diego; CA

Pfieffer JW, Jones JE (1979) *Reference Guide to Handbooks and Annuals*, Vol. i–vii. University Associates, San Diego; CA

Quinn F (1995) *The Principles and Practice of Nurse Education*, 3rd edn. Chapman and Hall, London

Race P (2000) *500 Tips on Group Learning*, Kogan Page, London

Schank MJ (1990) Wanted: nurses with critical thinking skills. *J Cont Educ Nurs* **21**(2): 86–89

Thoresen P (1972) Defence mechanisms in groups. Cited in: Pfeiffer W, Jones JE. *The Annual Handbook for Group Facilitators*. University Associates, La Jolla; CA

Tiberius R (1999) *Small Group Teaching: A Trouble- Shooting Guide*. Kogan Page, London

Tuckman BW (1965) Developmental sequences in small groups. *Psychol Bull* **63**: 384–99

Wallace D (1996) Experiential learning and critical thinking in nursing. *Nurs Stand* **10**: 31; 43–47

Watkins P (2001) *Mental Health Nursing: The Art of Compassionate Care*. Butterworth-Heinemann, Oxford

Wilkinson J, Wilkinson C (1996) Group discussions in nursing education: a learning process. *Nurs Stand* **10**: 44; 46–47

5

Creative solutions? Face the fear of academic essay writing! You really can do it!

The aim of this chapter is to reassure and empower students, suggesting ways to equip themselves for the challenges of assessment in mental health nursing by facing the fear of essay writing. The essay is an important academic tool for assessment. Much has been written and discussed in relation to essay writing (Beeson, 1993; 1996; Booth, 1996; Hamill, 1999; Redman, 2002; Shermis et al, 2001), by providing positive ways to write essays. However, in order to encourage students to see essay writing as a positive learning experience, the author suggests a new method called creative solutions, which is based on his own experiences and positive results with students. This approach should prove useful as more nursing courses move to degree and post-graduate level.

Introduction

> 'I stare at the blank page and think I can't do it, I don't know how to start and then I leave it, and it's no easier when I get back.'

> 'I've got children and a husband, it's like a juggling game trying to find time.'

> 'I have coffee, chat to friends, I'd paint walls do anything not to have to do it.'

> 'I cried, I was so scared of failing and I have worked so hard to get here.'

I am writing this chapter in this way, primarily because of the encouragement I was given by my own teachers. The most positive was on an evening course in psychology in 1986, before I went to university as a mature student to study. I found writing very difficult and I was anxious as a student and preoccupied about failing. One teacher was very encouraging, which is what I needed. It was clear she loved teaching psychology, and helping students to learn. It was the essay writing and the feedback that helped me most to progress. When my essays were returned to me, there were always careful notes and positive comments no matter what the grade. You really can do it she said, and with hard work I began to believe this and started on the road to success. In many ways, I am only putting forward the best encouragement to you from the teachers on my own journey in educating myself. You really can do it and it can be fun!

Watching students succeed is incredibly rewarding and satisfying to me as a teacher. It is even more rewarding in mental health nursing because we share a common interest. Students have helped me to develop and grow immensely. I find a personal approach with students and a passion for the subject area can be a great motivator. Positive encouragement is essential for the success of all students, as they may be very fearful and doubtful about their own abilities and capabilities. It is a major hurdle that can hold many truly gifted people back.

A knowledge of the psychology of the person provides much needed inspiration to work effectively with a wide variety of personalities and abilities, in and outside the classroom. Students have to battle and juggle with different demands on their time and receive little positive feedback in practice. Lecturers and teachers have a finite amount of time available, and their talents are not always valued. To facilitate students, a teacher needs to be approachable and practical in order to create motivation, co-operation and a positive and structured approach to learning. Seminars, tutorials, workshops and group work are all part of the support structure needed for students. Many universities have a writing skills support facility, and teachers can refer students for general and specific support with writing skills. However, many student are shy about admitting the need for help and some only arrive when they have failed an assignment.

'In nursing, it's rare for anyone to tell you you have done anything right, so if you get through you think, well it must have been alright; you just aim to pass.'

(Student)

'I failed an essay, and then I had another assignment to do and I was on placement; I felt like pulling my hair out, and then I felt insecure as the tutor that marked the essay wasn't available'.

(Student)

'We read the guidelines in class, I was afraid to say I didn't understand, everyone else seemed fine with it. I have learned since that you really have to ask questions.'

(Student)

One of the most daunting experiences about undertaking a course at a university is not so much the architecture, but getting used to an academic culture. Whether you come from Ireland or South Africa, at some point you will have to grapple with essays and assessments of one kind or another. You only have to overhear conversations with students to identify that writing an essay is seen as a fearful task rather than a positive learning experience. This is an important place to start if students are to feel motivated. An understanding of the psychology of learning and the individual student is important. In order to be effective as a teacher, we need to employ creative solutions and help students combat their fears about essay writing. Sometimes this may mean an English Language International Support Programme and referral to more specific resources. Creative solutions is one method of combining an understanding of the person with the task to be learned, namely, essay writing.

Creative solutions: a step-by-step model

The main components of creative solutions are facing the fear, energising, motivating and getting started, understanding what is expected, written and oral instructions, group work and coaching, the nuts and bolts, feedback and reworking, spelling out the standards, and getting results.

From the start, teacher and student expectations need to be discussed in a group, themes need to be identified and any mismatch with students dealt with. This model can be used with a group to maximise benefits from sharing with other students. This can be further developed by tutorials and workshops tailored to issues that can be dealt with in the group and individually. Such a method helps to prevent students failing assignments, and is best viewed as a preventative measure, eliminating much of the fear associated with essay writing.

Stage One: Facing the fear

You have to be a student to understand how fear and anxiety can stop you from beginning an essay; to know how crippling this anxiety can be. Many students say they do anything rather than knuckle down to their work. This is why having a coach is important. You have to become this coach yourself and with the right training you can do it. I know what this anxiety is like because I have experienced it myself. As a result of that experience I am putting forward a method that works. It is a combination of work between the teacher and student. Creative solutions is not just about getting started, although that is a significant step, but is also about keeping to the task and getting results.

Getting started begins by encouraging students to talk openly about their fears concerning essay writing. At this point, each student needs to describe his or her own particular fear. Previously, writers have talked about writers' block and many have suggested ways to relieve it (Flowers, 1981; Pagana, 1989). However, few talk about the management of the fear. Authors suggest just writing anything so you get started, not worrying about grammar, references, and spelling. However, the fear is much more intense and broader than these factors. It seems to be about fear of failure, lack of confidence, feeling isolated and lonely, fear of separation, past negative experiences with learning, and a lack of self-esteem, particularly in relation to the task of writing.

It may also be due to students feeling that anything they write will not reach the required standard and so avoid trying to do it, while others want the essay to be perfect straight away. So, in a real way, managing the fear creatively holds the key to achieving success. Working with a teacher and a group provides an anchoring support for students. Preparation at the start talks students through the process, and detailed feedback and sharing ensure support is real, while their fears are discussed openly, challenged and understood. Students need to feel supported and have a clear structure.

Breaking down the task of the essay into smaller components can be helpful, even if students do not follow the same sequences or steps. Such an approach leads to increased confidence and a feeling of control (Northedge, 1992; Booth, 1996). It is important to examine the title given for the essay and be clear of what is required. This is a pre-requisite for writing a good essay. Highlighting key words or phrases is useful in identifying the style, structure, and direction of the essay. For example, the word 'discuss' could mean to break down an issue into its component parts, discuss and evaluate these with examples, show how these inter-relate with reference to known authorities, as well as including one's own views (Rowntree, 1988).

This is important, as many students need to learn to plan their work using associated skills individually and collectively. It is essential for students to learn that a critical approach is required from the start in all academic writing, and the lack is a major weakness in many essays. Obtaining key references is another important step, and students need to book time in the library to learn how to use CD-Rom databases. Other ways of obtaining references include looking through newspaper articles, using the Internet and reading specific journals. Some guiding questions are useful, and as you check the literature, further references surface as you read in depth. You should organise themes that have emerged from the literature. Note taking is very important and students will need help with this in drawing out the main themes from articles and learning organisational skills.

The purpose of taking notes is to increase your knowledge about a subject, put concepts together and instil information in your minds, aid concentration when reading, provide a basis for revision in the future, integrate an assignment in relation to its parts, and store and organise information. The contents of your notes should include the key points of the subject, logical pictures, any important references, space for adding relevant examples, quotations, or additional material you might come across later. It is useful to note keywords as you read or listen. There are various styles of note taking, from linear notes to pattern notes (Gillett, 1990).

Accessing references online via a computer is a useful skill to learn early in any nursing course. Students should be aware of their deadline, so that they can allocate sufficient time to finding the key references. Sometimes, tutors have references available for specific assignments. Students need to learn to be selective in their choice of literature for each essay and this selectivity is necessary for teachers, too, thus ensuring that students are clear about what is required.

Support is essential, especially as many students are coming back into education, perhaps after considerable time out. Confidence needs fostering and friends and family need to learn to be supportive (study needs to fit in with your existing lifestyle). Other support comes from your personal tutor, lecturers, fellow students, other colleagues, or a writing support unit. Reading, too, can be developed and improved (Redman, 2002; Rowntree, 1988).

Stage Two: Energising, motivation and getting started

Energising, motivation and getting started is part of facing the fear. Positive sharing in a group is useful in order to foster motivation and encouragement. From the start, students need to be encouraged to be creative in challenging and finding solutions to their own fears. This can be done in a systematic way with the teacher as a facilitator. Part of this is demystifying the process of writing and placing it into everyday life that students can relate to. This requires the teacher to discuss problems experienced by the student in order to develop a clear understanding of what is preventing him/her from being successful in writing an essay. Reasons could stem from past experiences at school, where individuals may have had negative experiences with learning writing skills.

After this, a clear indication of what is expected in an academic essay needs to be outlined. Some students feel relieved and others have questions. Facing the fear requires that each student describes their fear, defines it, and plans a way of facing it, as part of a group and individually. This experience will identify common fears of all the students and how creative solutions can help conquer the fear of writing. Part of these solutions could involve setting up a buddy system. At this point, students become aware that they are one of many with fears about writing essays and, as a result, no longer feel isolated. Each person is encouraged to think about and draw resources together and, even before putting pen to paper, students will feel more supported with a much clearer focus on the task.

Stage Three: Written and oral instructions

In this part of the model, the teacher can act as a helper and inform students of what is expected in an academic essay. This could be in the form of written and oral instruction. Following instructions, it is always useful to check that students understand what is being explained before progressing, as some find it hard to ask questions. It is important to inform students that redrafting essays is part of the writing craft, and that reading and writing go hand in hand. Simply put, an essay comprises an introduction, the main body of the text and a conclusion

The Introduction   You need to identify how you are going to approach the essay. There is no definitive approach, but it is vital to justify why you are going to proceed with the essay in this particular way. You need to specify what aspects you will be dealing with and why. It might be useful to comment on the main topic of the essay, what you understand by it, how you interpret the terms, the main issues you will address and the assumptions you wish to make. You also need to identify how you are going to structure your essay.

The Main Body   This is the main part of your essay. However, do avoid the temptation of just writing everything you know on a set topic and making it purely descriptive in content. You need to deal with the main points. If you are not sure what these are, you need to obtain clarification rather than waste time. These points need to follow a rational argument and logical sequence. You need to justify these with relevant examples. Conflicting evidence should also be considered. Each issue you have introduced earlier can form a paragraph and for each new subject a new paragraph is needed. All references should be correctly cited.

The Conclusion   This should bring your whole argument together and summarise all the points you have made in your essay. It is a summing up of ideas and allows you to highlight implications, future trends or areas for further research. Conclusions are usually longer than the introduction section, but the quality of the content is a more important consideration.

Unlike other approaches, the teacher will coach each student not only on writing techniques and structure, which are essential, but also content organisation, sentence and paragraph construction. At this stage, the group can be assigned various writing tasks to explore levels of writing skill. The group is used as a resource, so some students can assist others as soon as they are deemed proficient. At this stage, the teacher can show sample essays as a guide, but only to students.

Stage Four: Group work and coaching: getting results

The group will become a resource and students will learn to work together, encouraged by the teacher. Students will also work independently after having instruction on reading and note taking. Improved essay results can be built on following preparation of each individual student by giving detailed feedback. Identify skills from previous learning.

Diagnose and describe the strengths and any problems experienced with each student. Identify new essay skills to develop with specific input. Identify new essay writing skills required using strengths identified from previous work as a base-line.

Written and oral instructions:

- Example of essays
- What is your standard

  New standard of how to write in general, and later in depth. Students are advised to read written instructions for their essay. These are checked after the teacher has gone through them verbally checking out any ambiguities with students. Following this, a learning contract is used to identify specific learning and a developmental plan of how this is to be achieved can then be drawn up.

The nuts and bolts, feedback and reworking, spelling out the standards and getting results:

- Contract for learning
- Developmental Plan

  This plan defines specific exercises for student, and the agreed level of intervention basic, moderate, or intensive. **Basic** means a very small amount of intervention by the teacher where the student is able and competent. The **intermediate** stage is where the student continues to need support in relation to structure and critical analysis. The **intensive** stage means providing a detailed tutorial and writing skills support for the student. The level of support is diagnosed and agreed by the teacher and student, then an agreed contract is drawn up with the student for dealing with the development of essay writing skills.

Then follows, for each person, a diagnosis of the individual fear he or she has. Fears are discussed and strategies put in place, which includes: tutorials, support, seminars, workshops, and referral to writing skills if needed. All students need to use previous learning as a means of building confidence. Students are encouraged to bring in essays in a folder to examine the strengths and weaknesses of previous work.

This can be used as a baseline to identify the need for new essay writing skills. Strategies to ensure progress can be put in place when students are clear who is there to help them and how the structure works in practice. They can compare new essay writing with previous work. Examples of essays are important for students to learn from and be clear about the standard required and their own personal standard. A Learning Contract identifies the student-specific goals and a developmental plan is a longer term plan of learning between student and teacher in learning essay writing skills. It also outlines how this will be achieved and what level of intervention will be required. If the student requires more help, it can be asked for and, equally, if the teacher considers more help is needed, additional support may be recommended.

The 'how' section will be explored in depth as part of the coaching of students; for example:

- how to create an argument
- the use of headings
- paragraph construction
- grammar
- the use of references
- defining terms
- using narratives
- sentence construction
- what is required in the essay
- understanding the essay title
- gaining control of essay content
- understanding essay guidelines
- working to the guidelines
- what is analysis
- critical thinking
- focussing the essay
- conclusion
- referencing.

The main body
- Establishing a valid argument
- facts
- academic writing style
- conclusion.

Resources
These include:
- teacher
- friends
- writing workshops
- self-help exercises
- feedback
- tutorials
- previous essays in a folder so that the student can see improvements or reasons for not improving.

Development Plan: How to do an essay

1. **Intensive**: step-by-step;

2. **Moderate**: requiring some input defined and agreed;

3. **Basic input**: checking over essay, references, argument, some feedback to alterations.

The main components to success in becoming a mental health nurse not only requires the student to acquire and develop clinical skills while on placements, but also academic writing skills. However, motivation is a key factor, and creative solutions offer a step-by-step approach to first gaining the confidence to try and then learning from structured support and feedback.

Such an approach creates solutions for the student and reduces the anxiety of learning, so that the only thing left is success. Many students who only aim for a pass mark may fail. Creative solutions require effort and time from students and their tutor, but the results make it worthwhile. Reduce your anxiety in academic essay writing by having the support that will get you through. Make writing a positive experience. Anxiety and fear can all be in the past, if you manage your fear with Creative Solutions using an effective, individual plan.

References

Beeson SA (1996) The effect of writing after reading on college nursing students' factual knowledge and synthesis of knowledge. *J Nurs Educ* **35**(6): 258–63

Beeson SA (1993) The effect of writing after reading on college nursing students' factual knowledge and synthesis of knowledge. The University Of North Carolina. PhD Unpublished Thesis.

Booth Y (1996) Writing an academic essay: a practical guide for nurses *Br J Nurs* **5**(16): 995–9

Flowers S (1981) Madman, architect, carpenter, judge: Roles and the writing process. *Language Arts* **58**: 834–6

Gillett H (1990) *Study Skills: A Guide for Healthcare Professionals*. Section 2.2 Managing your time. London South Bank Polytechnic, Distance Learning Centre, London

Hamill C (1999) Academic essay writing in the first person: a guide for undergraduates. *Nurs Stand* **13**(44): 38–40

Northedge A (1992) *The Good Study Guide*. Open University Press, Milton Keynes

Pagana K (1989) Writing strategies to demystify publishing. J *Contin Educ Nurs* **20**(2): 58–63

Redman P (2002) *Good Essay Writing*. Sage, London

Rowntree D (1988) *Learn How to Study: A Guide for Students of All Ages*. MacDonald, London

Shermis MD, Mzumara HR, Oslon J, Harrington S (2001) *On-line Grading of Student Essays: PEG Goes on the World Wide Web*. Journal Article: 2002-02555-005

6

Being a mental health nurse: A brief snapshot?

T his chapter will offer students a brief snapshot to explore what it is like to be a mental health nurse based on the author's experience as a mental health nurse, teacher, and therapist. Insight and experiences of nurses themselves in clinical practice in acute mental health settings will also be outlined. An acute mental health setting is the area of a hospital or a mental health unit where a person with a mental health problem is admitted. The mental health nurse has a central role in the admission process. Anxiety and depression will be used as working examples to illustrate basic components of caring for a person with a mental health problem.

Anxiety and depression

Can you remember a situation or time when you felt anxious? Have you ever been so terrified your stomach is in knots and you wanted to cry? Have you ever felt scared because you felt you would lose control? Have you ever been scared of public speaking, entering a room of strangers, being unable to express how you feel, being able to say no or being able to ask for what you want or need? Do you continuously have negative or obsessive thoughts going round your head? Are you over sensitive or irritable? Do you get things out of perspective? Anxiety and depression eats away at people's confidence and self-esteem turning them into a shell of the person they are meant to be, reducing their quality of life and unable to enjoy living or taking risks.

A serious aspect of these problems is that it can destroy the quality of relationships and distort a person's personality. It is not unusual for people with such problems to want to end relationships abruptly, often because they are finding it hard to cope themselves and manage their anxious and depressed feelings. Part of my role as a nurse and therapist is to teach people how to tackle anxiety and depression and, in so doing, understand themselves better. The relationship between nurse/therapist and client is crucial. A skilled nurse or therapist can help a person to learn to cope better and can transform a person's daily life. As a therapist, I have to work skilfully with a person to show them I genuinely care about them, and gain their trust. I show them that there is another way to live and that they can beat anxiety and depression; but this takes time, investment and effort. Structure is an essential part of my work. As a therapist, I am in control of the environment and it is far different from working on an acute ward.

Learning to cope

Whether you are on a ward or not, an important part of the role of the nurse or therapist is to help the person to develop stronger coping strategies. It is important to gain an understanding and appreciation of how people with anxiety feel. A mental health nurse can help a user to learn new coping skills to deal with his or her anxiety and depression. Nurses are familiar with being in a supportive role and offering reassurance. They realise that medication is not the answer on its own and each person is an individual. As a nurse and therapist, I have worked with people with anxiety and depression. They are often surprised that they can learn new ways of coping and they need constant reassurance and lots of support. You can appreciate how people's lives become ruled by fear and deep sadness. Every aspect of their life can be ruined, leading to low self-esteem, poor self-image, no confidence, sleep problems and, worst of all, feelings of uselessness and self-hate. There needs to be engagement with the user, and a therapeutic relationship. As a nurse, if you can have time to engage with users, they will learn much about themselves and, at the same time, you can learn through experience. The next section will briefly outline how to read the signs.

Reading the signs

Anxiety and depression have costs; in absence from work and, more importantly, in human suffering (Nolen-Hoeksema, 2001). It is the most prevalent mental health issue of our time (Stuart and Sundeen, 1997). Anxiety can range in severity from mild to panic attacks where the person feels completely out of control. Anxiety and depression often go together and such problems are very common (Klerman, 1987). Depressed feelings range from tiredness, lethargy, lack of motivation, and sleeplessness, to feeling hopeless and suicidal. Perhaps more difficult, is the ability for the person to recognise his/her problem as psychological and emotional, to know where to get help and to have the confidence to ask for it. It is not uncommon for individuals to avoid looking for help or to deny they have a problem at all. How should we, as nurses, care in acute settings? Ideally, mental health nursing will be about caring, empowering, teaching people life skills, coping skills and social skills for living. However, nurses in practice face a daunting reality, with many challenges. Like users, nurses need to feel valued and feel they have a future. They need a structured framework of hope. Users and their families need to be able to share their feelings with others and receive practical and skilled help. Medication will not teach new coping skills, or build self-esteem and that is why skilled mental health nurses are essential at every level of service provision. In acute settings, the reality for nurses is stark, challenging and needing serious attention from all stake holders in mental health. Most importantly, we must learn to invest in and value the expertise and experience of mental health nurses.

Valuing the experience and work of mental health nurses

It is timely that the work of mental health nurses in acute settings now takes centre stage. After all, this work is not solely about medical intervention and medication. Clearly, any snapshot will be limited in capturing much of the actual work of nurses in practice. The focus on acute mental health nursing is poignant given the increasing critical attention to lack of care provision in acute services in mental health in the UK (Gijbels, 1995; Rix *et al*, 1999; Rose, 2000; Sainsbury, 2002; 2001; 1998; 1997; Warner *et al*, 2000).

It is vital that the expertise and experience of mental health nurses are valued from the outset in promoting, delivering, and creating more effective and user friendly mental health services for users and their families (Hughes *et al*, 1996; Midence and Gamble, 1995; Oppong-Tutu and Price, 1997). It is important that mental health nursing care is not eroded or devalued by fanciful ideas or visions of other, more powerful professionals or politicians.

'The staffing levels, well... I don't want to go into it but... I wouldn't say I felt really, really scared, but I didn't feel safe on the ward.'

(Female student, 26-year-old)

'It's was like going in at the deep end, working on an acute mental health ward, but I learned more in the first few weeks after qualifying than I ever did as a student nurse.'

(Female student, 26-year-old)

'Morale is low sometimes because we can't do the job we are trained for, and patients are often at the lower end of the day's priorities and you are up for an early a shift the following day, which all leads to high levels of stress.'

(Staff Nurse)

'Yes I have read books, but being a mental health nurse is nothing like what you read about or see on television, I think we all know that most books are nothing like reality...in this kind of nursing you can't hide behind a uniform...you see people's lives in pieces... and over time the questions you get asked search every part of your soul...'

(Staff Nurse)

'When I first qualified, a few years ago, perhaps I could go along with 'pull your socks up' or 'things are not that bad' mentality.

But I am an experienced nurse now and I know that mental health problems, like depression and schizophrenia are much more complex than this. It is important to facilitate learning about nursing interventions for students and newly qualified staff. However, in practice there is hardly time for patients let alone staff and we are in a constant flux of change, I always feel guilty.'

(Staff Nurse)

'Some days I can't be bothered anymore, one shift can be so stressful I just go in do my shift and get out...there is really nothing glamorous about being a mental health nurse...then there are other days when I know that my approach made a difference, my contribution counted, but those are few.'

(Staff Nurse)

'Sometimes I feel like I have given all I can give as a person, but there is always another demand always someone wanting another piece of me...you have to work on a busy acute service to believe the intensity of the work...and the kind of emotional atmosphere.'

(Staff Nurse)

'I'm fortunate. I work with a great team in a new unit... I know it's not like an acute ward... I feel guilty as I know things are not so good for my colleagues.'

(Staff Nurse)

'I have children. It's my livelihood... I guess the reality is the conditions in this acute service are terrible, but I love the work with patients... the sad reality is we are all torn between other, non nursing activities...and sometimes I wonder if anyone really listens to us mental health nurses.'

(Staff Nurse)

The above quotes are part of a research study undertaken by the author, and give a sample of mental health nurses' diverse views of what it's like to be a mental health nurse in an acute setting. The study was similar in design to other nursing studies (Benner, 1985; Gijbels, 1995). Users' views also help to refocus our attention on the care they need and the everyday obstacles they face.

Mental health

'I think stigma is sometimes the cause of the isolation and loneliness that many people like ourselves find themselves in. Stigma arises from a lack of understanding and a lack of contact. If these problems were addressed, possibly at school, then maybe some headway could be made for future generations, if not for ourselves.'

(Service User)

'It took the psychiatrist from 1972 to 1990 to get my diagnosis right, so I was thirty years without a diagnosis at all. I first went to hospital in 1968 and was told I was a hypochondriac... I was lost in the system and it took until 1993 for a locum to tell me, what I already knew, that I was a fast-cycler and should have been on carbamazepine and lithium combined. There, that's professional help for you.'

(Hill *et al*, 1996)

The above is a user account about the stigma of having a mental health problem, and another person's experience about being diagnosed with a bipolar mood disorder where the person may have periods of over activity, hence the expression 'fast cycler'.

In the same survey, community mental health nurses (CPNs) were positively evaluated in comparison to general practitioners, who were seen to be poorly informed about mood disorders.

Key terms

In mental health nursing, there are a number of key terms; working definitions given in *Chapter 4* will provide a useful start. (Thomas *et al*, 1997; Townsend, 1996). This is an introductory text and will only provide a snapshot for students who may be interested in following a career in mental health nursing.

In mental healthcare in hospital and the community, the person with a mental health problem is called the user, the client, the patient, etc. Nurses have many titles depending on their role and qualifications; a staff nurse, the mental health nurse, mental health worker, the community psychiatric nurse, clinical nurse specialist, nurse advisor, nurse consultant, therapist, etc. The prevalence of mental health problems is around one in every four families in the UK (Goldburg, 1995) and similar prevalence rates exist in the US (Nolen-Hoeksema, 2001). However, there is strong debate surrounding the influence of race and culture (Fernando, 2002).

Nursing skills

The skills mental health nurses have and employ are varied and can be broken down into therapeutic skills, which include: caring and comforting, interpersonal and counsel-ling, psychotherapeutic interventions, crisis intervention, family therapy, co-ordination and communication, teaching and management, control and restraint, administrative, IT, supervision, observational, advanced practice, advanced therapeutic, group work, advocacy, leadership, and skills specific to drug administration; and knowledge on trust policies, which include: fire prevention, and health and safety. There is much obstruction in maintaining, developing and using these skills in acute settings, sometimes in impoverished environments. (Gijbels, 1995; Sainsbury, 2002; Sainsbury, 1998).

Settings and client groups

Mental health nurses work in a variety of settings and with a variety of client groups. These include: dealing with child and adolescents, adult, older people, behavioural problems, forensic, rehabilitation, eating disorders, community projects, etc., and back-to-work schemes. As a mental health nurse, we deal with the effects of many emotional and psychological problems, from anxiety, depression, eating disorders, autism, and schizophrenia, to common phobias, behavioural problems, sexual, emotional or physical abuse, various alcohol and addictive disorders, etc. Some authors have integrated texts that offer clear ideas in working with enduring mental health problems (Gamble and Brennan, 2000).

Research

Research in mental health nursing has increased over the last 20 years. In this genre, research has focussed on a number of areas, in particular, community psychiatric nursing, nurse as therapist, etc., while the role mental health nurses perform in the traditional hospital-based settings appears to have taken a back seat (Gijbels, 1995; Keltner, 1985). The interest in acute mental health care, rather than mental health nursing, has recently been resurrected and is in the spotlight (Sainsbury, 1998).

Mental health nursing

Stigma levelled at users with mental health problems, is also levelled at mental health nurses. This is sometimes translated into a kind of deep seated fear or disrespect for qualified mental health nurses, who are often viewed as 'not proper nurses' by others in the nursing profession.

Perhaps there is still an irrational fear of contamination in parts of the adult nursing fraternity. This prejudicial view in adult nursing might be part of the sanitisation process instilled by figures, such as Florence Nightingale, where hygiene was the order of the day. However, according to historical accounts, Florence Nightingale took to her bed for weeks at a time during her life without any known physical cause (Nolan, 1993). So perhaps she was not as infallible as people have suggested. Hygiene being the order of the day and adult nursing being viewed as clean and proper, then is the work of mental health nurses dirty?

Mental health nursing, although valued by many people, continues to be viewed with significant criticism and stigma. Many have indicated that over the last twelve years mental health nursing is in a 'wilderness' (Burnard, 1990), and others suggest that, on the one hand, it is a medical support system and on the other, emphasise, in part, its interpersonal basis (Barker, 1990).

Moving from medical to psychosocial orientation

Other writers have indicated that that a shift was taking place from a medical to a psychosocial orientation and even referred to a mental health nursing paradigm (Adams, 1991). In 2002, there is little evidence of a mental health nursing paradigm and there continues to be much debate surrounding how best to deliver care in under-resourced and under-staffed mental health services (Campbell, 2000; Sainsbury, 1998).

Mental health nursing is defined in different ways in relation to therapeutic relationships (Barker, 1990; Watkins, 2001). Some authors focus on the role (Peplau, 1987), others on the orientation, and on the approach and underlying ethos of the profession (Adams, 1991).

Back to basics

The hallmarks of effective mental health nursing is about relationships, which need to focus on closeness, attentiveness, supportiveness and flexibility (Altschul, 1972), a sentiment echoed by (Barker, 1999). Annie Altschul can speak with some authority, as she herself was a nurse and a professor, an expert mental health nurse, and a person with depression.

It is clear that in order to achieve closeness to a person, there has to be time, an appropriate culture of caring and objective and instrumental tools to make that not only possible, but sustainable. Mental health nurses in acute settings often feel challenged in relation to forging therapeutic time with users; in developing closeness, attentiveness, supportiveness, and flexibility. If we are unable to deliver such qualities to users, it would appear that mental health nurses in acute settings are being deskilled and users deprived of meaningful therapeutic relationships.

Current practice

Currently, many mental health nurses in practice speak about mental health nursing as an ever changing set of tasks, with increased intensity of work, decreased quality of time with users, changing needs and priorities, new reports and legislation. More speak about mental health nursing as some distant ideal, others say mental health nursing in hospital settings is left behind, has moved back or is moving back more and more to custodial care, and dominated by form filling or other non-nursing activities. In the community, there is much more scope, diversity and investment (Gamble and Brennan, 2000), yet what will happen to nurses and users in acute mental health services. We need to find acute solutions (Sainsbury, 2001).

Modern approaches in acute settings often incorporate initial assessment on admission, which includes what can be referred to as a minimum data set. It is not uncommon for a nurse and doctor to undertake an admission together. Care needs to be taken that nurses clearly identify nursing, not medical needs. However, the pacing of each admission varies widely and in practice not all admissions are completed immediately. Staff nurses try to manage the situation of the person being admitted with what is already happening on the ward. If the person is crying and very distressed, the staff nurse has to manage the situation, as well as managing other staff and clients. Multi-tasking has become the norm in acute mental health settings. As a result, staff nurses often speak of being distracted or unable to complete tasks properly.

This draws on the staff nurses' ability to manage, communicate, prioritise and deliver in often stressful situations. It must also be appreciated that not all persons being admitted are calm or want to be admitted. Some admissions may take hours, involving the support of other staff who are often very experienced and skilled.

However, in some situations, it may be more difficult as there are relatively few staff or experienced staff available. Some of the information for a minimum data set includes background generic information, such as, age, gender, referral source, medication, next of kin, etc. Some information may seem unnecessary to the unqualified eye, but when a person leaves an acute ward, they may continue to be a danger to themselves or others. You can then understand why a full description of the person is essential.

A physical examination is part of the admission process and includes taking blood pressure, pulse and respiration, usually by the doctor. Other medical tests are often identified. It is also necessary to list what the person brought with him/her and items that need to be taken away and stored for safekeeping.

In forensic units and some acute units with specific policies, there may be drug screening and a detailed search to ensure the person is alcohol and drug free. On admission, an interview continues to be the main method of data collection, often incorporating an admission pack. An admission pack could incorporate nursing models, such as those of Roper Logan and Tierney, Peplau, and Orem, assessment schedules and, in some cases, a specific philosophy of care.

A brief description of tasks will be considered to give an insight into aspects of what mental health nurses do in practice. It is important to state that many units, including community and outreach teams, have their own culture and often have more contact with patients than clinical psychologists or psychiatrists (Midence and Gamble, 1995), and community psychiatric nurses (CPNs) could have an important role in training other health professionals (Leff and Gamble, 1995).

Verbal handover, administration and observation

On an acute mental health ward, the main communication tool continues to be the handover towards the end of each shift. In summary, the staff nurse in charge of the shift on a ward will feed back to the nursing team issues arising in respect of individual clients. Some planning for the future is often discussed, including likely interventions, the exact number of clients on the ward, and others on leave.

Many wards have a report that is completed and documents movements or changes with clients and staff. The style and order varies significantly, depending on the ward or unit, and some staff prefer to supplement this report with care plans or programmes of care. Some units share the responsibility for a period of time and may reorder or prioritise the care. Methods employed by nurses can be complex and detailed, so notes are a necessity. Aspects of care should be checked and rechecked, as sometimes the behaviour of a client needs specialist observation, monitoring and practical hands on intervention.

Observations, such as one-to-one observation, can only be carried out by a qualified mental health nurse who has the specialist training and knowledge. During this observation, the client has to be less than an arm's distance away at all times and is very invasive. Reports for courts are also written by qualified nurses and it is not unusual for nurses to be called upon as consultants or expert witnesses in their field of mental health.

For the purposes of this chapter, the handover is defined as a place where staff come together, give a verbal account, and discuss aspects of care and staffing at the beginning and end of each shift. In some units, there is often a friendly and social aspect to this, especially where staff know each other and are familiar with care practices. Key aspects of care are allocated to individual nurses and nursing assistants, as well as key observation rotas and specialist care. Breaks may also be agreed and choice is often a part of care where people may negotiate certain tasks and care. The style of handovers vary, some being more democratic and others more authoritative or ritualistic.

There is usually a ward diary, which may be in a book or on a ward computer, where information about appointments and the activities of each day is kept. If you are co-ordinating the shift, it will be your responsibility to read this and deal with all items given priority. You need to be aware that some wards have a board where key points are outlined for staff, including who is taking care of a given client and times of observation checks and breaks. Abbreviations may be used for confidentiality.

As a staff nurse, you must be conversant with various policies, including fire precautions and drills, and health and safety. Knowledge of ward policies and trust policies is essential and learning how to supervise junior staff and liaise with other professionals is a basic requirement.

Safety and dealing with a crisis

Another important aspect of being a staff nurse is learning what to do in a crisis or emergency, and how to deal with your own mistakes and those of others. Learning to manage situations and other staff takes time and often the support of colleagues. Administering medication is still a central aspect of the daily work of mental health nurses. Knowledge about specific drugs and their action is part of the course, as are procedures for injections, controlled drugs and the Mental Health Act.

Multi-tasking

Currently, mental health nursing requires a person in an acute mental healthcare setting to have the ability to learn how to multi-task and at the same time communicate effectively with, and be responsive to, clients and staff. The role is split between managing, communicating, organising, supervising, leading, facilitating, administrating and, at the same time, trying to be therapeutic.

An important insight for student nurses is the experience of admission and its effects. It is probably the most frightening experience for a person, already in severe psychological distress, to be admitted to a mental health unit, however modern or friendly. Users talk of many feelings surrounding admission, for example, being anxious, powerless, helpless, ashamed, confused, frightened, angry, in disbelief, relieved, feeling imprisoned, feeling punished, etc.

Like any clinician or professional, student nurses need information and insights into practice and the diversity of the work in this field. A case study will be employed to highlight the impact of the admission process on an acute mental health ward. Anxiety is a common mental health problem (WHO, 1992), and will be used to highlight some aspects of the practical day-to-day work of a mental health nurse on an acute ward.

Admission to an acute mental health unit: Case Study

John Mullins is 46 years old and has been married to Tracey for 20 years. They have one child, Michael aged 15 years. After leaving school, John worked in a large petrochemical company and is now one of the directors. He has never experienced difficulties in forming relationships and has always had an active social life. In the last year, he has gained promotion and since then has gradually developed feelings of inadequacy, low-self esteem, self-doubt and is having difficulty in making decisions. His colleagues have tried to reassure him that his work is up to his usual standard.

Despite these assurances, he finds himself unable to stop worrying. John was treated by his general practitioner for three months, making little progress, before being referred to a consultant psychiatrist. Following the consultation, he agreed to an admission for assessment and is at present resident on an integrated acute ward within a large general hospital.

The initial action would be to explore the basis of his anxiety and, when this is achieved, appropriate interventions could be employed. These could include familiarising John with the environment and dealing with any uncertainty by answering as many questions as possible. It is important to interview the client and significant people in his life to clarify their perceptions, expectations and personal details; observing actions, interactions, self-rating scales, and life skills; collecting relevant data, such as reports compiled by other health professionals.

All these processes form part of a nursing assessment used by mental health nurses in practice. The feelings that John is expressing need to be accepted by the nurse. It is important that the nurse fosters independence rather than dependence. Such dependence can be avoided by acknowledging the reality of his concerns and offering to look at available options and strategies with him. Some nurses and therapists find it useful to draw a diagram to encourage engagement of clients in understanding what is happening to them and helping them to develop strategies with which to cope. Depersonalisation and the fostering of the 'sick role' is often the result of admission to hospital. With a perception such as this, John would believe 'I am sick, you are the helpers'.

As a result, the focus of nursing care would be more concerned with doing to, rather than doing with, and this is how dependence is fostered. When a person is anxious, the physiological response is a state of readiness: the fight or flight response. Due to the release of the hormone, adrenaline, specific physiological changes occur. There is also a change in the individual's level of arousal and, therefore, a higher risk that this will increase the chances of stimuli being misinterpreted. The nurse has specific responsibilities in relation to John's admission. The requirement is to maintain the respect and dignity of the person, given that many people feel very vulnerable. This can be helped if the nurse maximises the client's involvement and independence.

The interview

An important aspect of a nursing assessment is conducting interviews with John and those individuals significant to him in his life. A great deal of relevant information can be gained in these interviews. Also important at this stage is clarifying John's perception of the problem, together with the expectations of him and his family.

Interviews need to be conducted in a quiet comfortable room and in a sensitive manner. Interview skills are developed through interpersonal skills training and, directly, in practice. It is essential that the interview creates a safe and relaxed atmosphere, and to convey your concern, interest and involvement. Such interviews can, at times, be very emotional and it is important to recognise which questions to pursue, which to ignore, and how long the duration of the interview should be. An experienced nurse will make these decisions promptly. People frequently cry and the relatives might need reassurance themselves. If the client is very distressed, his/her welfare is paramount, and long pauses and the closure of the interview are part of the course.

Frequently, nurses and doctors are flexible and understanding in these situations. Nurses are often asked questions, such as, 'How long will John be in hospital for?' An honest answer is best. It is impossible to say how long this could be until a comprehensive assessment is carried out, would be the correct answer. When one member of a family is admitted, it has important and, sometimes profound, effects on the dynamics of the family.

John has, up to now, managed his own life; he has managed the finances of the home. His wife may feel at a loss, abandoned and uncertain of the future due to John's admission. She may also experience feelings of loss, remorse, guilt and perhaps a degree of hostility. Such feelings could be displaced on to John and their child or the hospital and its staff. Nurses often experience this and, occasionally, feelings of blame. Alternatively, relatives can view nurses as providing hope for themselves and the client.

Therapeutic work, tasks and routines

Admission, assessment, therapeutic relationship, the nursing process, report writing, observation, attentiveness, checking observation, medication, meals, meetings, handover, supervision, care plans, allocation of duties and care, etc., are all part of a day in the life of a staff nurse. What is often forgotten is that many staff have young children and other responsibilities outside of work.

Nurses, experienced in working in an acute setting, will be subject to many demands and are familiar with endless activity, physical, emotional and mental. Staff unfamiliar with this area of work will not appreciate the reality of mental and physical exhaustion at the end of a shift and, in some cases, the need for apparently relentless, but necessary safety checks and routines.

Part of this tiredness is the hidden stress of staff nurses' responsibility for others who might self harm, abscond or create conflict, and the need to be in a state of ready alertness not, as many might think, relaxation. The process of admission is an important task and creates anxiety for most people involved. The reasons are numerous, but it is the responsibility of the nurse to allay anxiety as effectively as possible. Another important point in mixed-sex acute wards is that nurses have to deal with ethical issues in relation to privacy, safety, personal space, sexuality, and feelings of embarrassment.

Learning

'Experience with patients is the best learning tool, not reading a book.'

(Female student; 43-year-old)

The above quote echoes views held by many student nurses, staff nurses and practitioners about the value of direct experience with users or clients. However, experience alone will not necessarily create learning, and those in practice are not always able or equipped to teach. Contrary to what many believe (Peplau, 1987), a mental health nurse needs knowledge and skills (Altschul, 1972; Barker, 1999).

Like doctors, some nurses are viewed as better than others; some for their compassion, others for their knowledge. Perhaps a combination of the two is the most sought after by users and their families, judging on research on user perspectives in mental health (Hill *et al*, 1996). Effective teaching of mental health nursing is required at all levels in practice and at university.

Tools such as books and specialist research can inform, nurture and develop practice only if valued by managers and clinicians. Relevant theory and practice are essential to be a knowledgeable doer (Brooking, 1986; Brooking *et al*, 1992) and, increasingly, this must include primary care (WHO, 2001).

We learn different things in different schools and practice is but one school, university another. Critical thinking comes from many areas of our lives, for example, critical experiences—personal and professional, reading, reflection and practice. There will always be changes in theory and language, but we need to be careful that fashion is not exchanged for valuable nursing expertise.

The Masters of Hope

The skilled mental health nurse is without doubt the master of hope in historical terms and in practice, and has had to be resilient in the face of barbaric and inhumane care, and an institutional and outside world that can be hostile, cruel, ignorant, and lacking in human kindness. As a ward manager in mental health myself in London in the nineties, I observed how nurses continued to sacrifice much to maintain basic standards of care. Many patients have real fears that they will never come back to health when they are first admitted to a mental health unit. Such fear needs constant reassurance from the nurse and, sadly, some individuals have frequent re-admissions.

In human rights terms, we need to contemplate the plight of individuals and families affected by mental health problems. We must face the fact that the history of mental health care is evolving and, together, we must do all we can to develop better services for everyone.

Currently, we live in a time where human life seems to be constantly devalued. Economic and social changes have their consequences, often affecting mental health and psychological well-being. More than at any other time, we have problems that relate to a global refugee crisis, war, and tragedies that include the rising incidence of mental health problems in children. This is the global backdrop, but day-to-day issues, working in mental health units and the community is a real eye opener to the visitor.

It is a very humbling experience to visit and realise where and how we mental health nurses are trying to dispense acute nursing care in the UK. It is possible that many professionals look, but fail to see the degrading conditions in which individuals with mental health problems are treated. Lack of staffing resources often means that there can be little real leadership in acute care. Stigma of mental illness permeates not only lay beliefs, but also so called professional attitudes. It is strange that nurse colleagues could have such negative attitudes given the dreadful emotional and psychological distress that many mental health nurses work with day in and day out, particularly in acute settings.

'You are made to feel less important because you are following a mental health nursing course, it's not always spoken but when you come together with other adult nursing students it is evident that their opinions are far from positive.'

(Student; Year 3)

Perhaps of more concern is the environments of care, which do little to enhance the image of progress in mental health. Unlike clinical psychologists and psychiatrists, mental health nurses are there in the environment with clients over a twenty-four hour period. The mental health nurse is one of the greatest gifts a civilised society can have at its disposal and one that must be invested in for the welfare of all individuals needing effective mental health care. The work of mental health nurses focusses on a person who is vulnerable. Unlike other nursing disciplines that focus on the physical domain, mental health nursing requires the use of self in forming relationships between nurses and users. Such relationships require a high level of integrity and flexibility. More importantly, mental health nurses are special in the sense that they are allowed to see what is sacred to a person, to see a person when normal layers have been stripped away, damaged, and broken. But more than this, the user is given the power to be themselves and some hope of being restored to health or adapting to their situation.

Anthony Claire, a famous professor of psychiatry, has discussed how professionals may be viewed as healers and the patients as those to be healed. The reality is that healing can come from the experience of having a mental health problem, as many users of mental health services will testify (Heyman, 1995; Hill *et al*, 1996).

Psychiatrists, doctors, nurses, and psychologists are not immune to experiencing mental health problems themselves. User groups understand that experience of a mental health problem, such as depression for example, can be a very positive catalyst for change. The healer may be within and/or outside of the person.

Our mental and emotional lives are rich in many spheres, including the mental, spiritual, and psychological dimensions. Although you will hear people talk about holistic nursing, there remains a pervasive emphasis on the treatment of health as primarily being in the physical domain, often disempowering individuals. Every day, the study of mental health links the possibility that there is more than a tenuous link between the mind, body and spirit, albeit a difficult one for scientists to quantify empirically. Our perception of mental health has so often been undervalued in society and this is echoed in science, which seems to value genes more than people and cure more than caring.

It is timely and fitting to understand, respect and appreciate the very special and individual contribution of mental health nurses. In particular, their kindness, sensitivity and caring in often very difficult and challenging circumstances. Throughout history, they have championed hope in providing better care and treatments. It would be sad if mental health nurses with degrees are left to care in acute services, administering new ideas in run down and under-resourced settings.

What power has an educated work-horse, if they are simply left to hold the fort, to administer medication and count beds? There continues to be inequality in professional power between nursing and medicine, even though nurses are much better educated today. This is a serious issue, where the knowledge of the nurse is comparable to that of the doctor and what constitutes appropriate treatment remains a medical decision. Perhaps nurses will never be free to care if their knowledge of caring is not viewed positively. Ironically, the science of cure seems elevated despite its failure, in real terms, to cure mental health problems,such as schizophrenia, or truly identify cogent preventative strategies for suicide. The history of mental health nursing illustrates that, more than in any other profession, the mental health nurse has risen from virtual obscurity and oppression to being the master of hope for users in their care. For users, mental health nurses remain the unsung heroes of care.

References

Adams A (1991) Paradigms in psychiatric nursing. *Nursing* 4(35): 9–11

Altschul A (1972) *Patient-Nurse Interaction: A Study of Interaction Patterns in Acute Psychiatric Wards*. Churchill Livingstone, Edinburgh

Barker P (1999) Common sense caring. *Nurs Stand* 3(44): 22

Barker P (1990) The conceptual basis of mental health. *Nurse Educ Today* 10: 339–48

Benner M (1985) Intensive interviewing. In: Benner M, Brown J, Canter D, eds. *The Research Interview: Uses and Approaches*. Academic Press, London: 147–62

Brooking J, ed (1986) *Psychiatric Nursing Research*. J Wiley and Sons, Chichester

Brooking J, Ritter S, Thomas B, eds (1992) *A Textbook of Psychiatric and Mental Health Nursing*. Churchill Livingstone, Edinburgh

Burnard P (1990) Changes in theory, language and psychiatric nursing. *Nexus* 1(4): 18–21

Campbell P (2000) Absence at heart. *OpenMind*, 104: 14–15

Fernando S (2002) *Mental Health Race and Culture*, 2nd edn. Palgrave, Hampshire

Gamble C, Brennan G (2000) *Working with Serious Mental Illness: A Manual for Clinical Practice*. Balliere Tindall, London

Gijbels H (1995) Mental health nursing skills in an acute admission environment: Perceptions of mental health nurses and other professionals. *J Adv Nurs* 21(3): 460–65

Goldburg D (1995) The fields trials of the mental disorders section of ICD-10 designed for primary care in England. *Fam Pract* 12(4): 383–84

Heyman B (1995) *Researching User Perspectives on Community Healthcare*. Chapman and Hall, London

Hill RG, Hardy P, Shepherd G (1996) *Perspectives on Manic Depression: A Survey of the Manic Depression Fellowship*. The Sainsbury Centre for Mental Health, London

Hughes I, Hailwood R, Abbati-Yeoman J, Budd R (1996) Developing a family intervention service for serious mental illness: clinical observations and experiences. *J Ment Health* **5**(2): 145–59

Keltner N (1985) Psychotherapeutic management: a model for nursing practice. *Persp Psychiatr Care* **23**(4): 125–30

Klerman GL (1987) Psychiatric epidimiology and mental health policy. In: Levine S, Lilienfield A, eds. *Epidemiology and Health Policy*. Tavistock, New York: 227–64

Leff J Gamble C (1995) Training of community psychiatric nurses in family work for schizophrenia. *Int J Ment Health* **24**(3): 76–88

Midence K, Gamble C (1995) Family work and attitudes to schizophrenia. *Nurs Times* **290**: 12

Nolan P (1993) *A History of Mental Health Nursing*. Chapman and Hall, London

Nolen-Hoeksema S (2001) *Abnormal Psychology*, 2nd edn. McGraw Hill, Boston

Oppong-Tutu A, Price V (1997) Working with the mentally ill and their families. *Ment Health Nurs* **17**(4): 8–10

Peplau H (1987) Tomorrow's world. *Nurs Times* **83**(1): 29–32

Rix S, Beadsmore A, Shepherd G, Finch J (1999) *Standards for Acute Mental Health Services. Health Advisory Service*. Pavilion Publishing, Brighton

Rose D (2000) Do it yourselves. *Ment Health Care* **2**(5): 174–77

Sainsbury (2002) *Briefing Paper 16: Acute Inpatient Care for People with Mental Health Problems*. Sainsbury Centre for Mental Health, London

Sainsbury (2001) *The Capable Practitioner. A Framework and List of the Practitioner Capabilities Required to Implement the National Service Framework in Mental Health*. The Sainsbury Centre for Mental Health, London

Sainsbury (1998) *Briefing Paper 4: Acute Problems: A Survey of the Quality of Care in Acute Psychiatric Wards*. Sainsbury Centre for Mental Health, London:

Sainsbury (1997) *Pulling Together: The Future Roles and Training of Mental Health Staff*. Sainsbury Centre for Mental Health, London

Stuart GW, Sundeen SJ (1997) *Mental Health Nursing Principals and Practice*, UK edn. Mosby, London

Thomas B, Hardy B, Cutting P (1997) In: Stuart GW, Sundeen SJ, eds. *Mental Health Nursing Principles and Practice*, UK edn. Mosby, London

Townsend CR (1996) *Ecology: Individuals, Populations and Communities*. Blackwell Scientific, Oxford

Warner L, Rose D, Mackintosh G, Ford R (2000) Could this be you? Evaluating quality and standards of care in the inpatient psychiatric setting. *Ment Health Care* **4**(3): 89–92

Watkins P (2001) *Mental Health Nursing: The Art of Compassionate Care*. Butterworth-Heinemann, Oxford

WHO (2001) *Guide to Mental Health in Primary Care*. Royal Society of Medicines, London

WHO (1992) *ICD-10 Classification of Mental and Behavioural Disorders*. World Health Organization, Geneva

7

Looking after
your own mental health?

'I couldn't stop crying, but I didn't want to admit I wasn't coping... I am so exhausted... you just get used to being so anxious all the time... over the years, I've been hit... and sworn at so much... and degraded by patients... assaulted—they say it goes with the territory... no real support or support groups and if there were, we are too short of staff to attend anyway... it's a joke... who cares for the carers? We are nurses yes... but we have needs too, human needs like anyone else... I have two children; I go home exhausted... they want a mother not a shell... but you see I am often too tired to talk to or give them the attention they require. More and more I need my space to relax... in reality the only relaxation I get is when I have the bathroom door locked and I am in the bath.'

(Lesley, Staff Nurse)

Nursing seems to be a window on caring that looks out to others. Yet on closer inspection perhaps we ought to be teaching nurses about balance and knowledge, about caring for themselves first. For to give too much can be detrimental for one's own health and possibly the health of others. There is a need for a revolution in mental health nursing to refocus the object of caring to self first and then to others.

Ironically, the title of this chapter indicates that we can look after our own mental health but, sadly, the facts indicate otherwise and there is a growing concern for the health and well-being of mental health professionals (Hiscott and Connop, 1990; Laryea, 2002). Humans are social animals, which is why people with few social networks are more vulnerable to mental health problems in the first place (Blacker and Clare, 1987). Many students would agree that emotional and mental health is dependant on friends, family, partners and other support mechanisms. Friends are so important to how we feel on a day-to-day basis. It is essential that we include emotional health as part of mental health.

As students, you need to learn how to make new friends, how to settle into university, and how to take care of yourself. For younger students, this may be a new found independence. Others may feel homesick. Single parents have important practical needs to be met in order to take up the course. Mature students have financial concerns, and sometimes feel guilty leaving the children. There can be stress between couples and the added strain of being a student does end some relationships. Students do experience anxiety and depression (Merrell, 2001); furthermore, there are students who underestimate the demands made on them, failing to recognise that ordinary experiences and changes can place huge pressures on their mental well being. So what do we need to do in order to cope more positively and take care of our own mental health?

Valuing ourselves

It is amazing the good one person can do, and students can bring so much joy and happiness sometimes, by just being there. Each student is important and you do not stop being important when you qualify as a nurse. It is vital that you appreciate who you are as a person not just as a nurse. Many experienced nurses have to take care of the staff as well as the users, and this is a real strain. Doctors and clinical psychologists can be far removed from the experiences of nurses managing a shift on an acute ward. However, it is clear that nurses are valued for what they can do for others and, in some cases, undervalued as people.

We need to value not only ourselves more, but also those around us who nurture us. In the caring world, we need to support each other, irrespective of professional background. If we stop valuing people whose job it is to care, they will be unable or unmotivated to continue caring to the same degree. Some people feel very isolated in their caring role and lack social support, themselves.

This kind of self-realisation is essential at some point in your life, so you first value yourself and can then take good care of yourself and others. Valuing yourself is not selfish. How did we learn to take care of ourselves? Who were the role models? Perhaps we need to relearn some of these skills. It should be an essential part of any educational course in mental health nursing, to build respect, confidence and self-esteem. It is sad but true that some individuals never really value themselves, and others have an overwhelming need to be needed. Such behaviour leads to burnout. If you are a manager, it is crucial to understand how each person copes with stress so that support can be tailored effectively. Love and hope are two of the most central aspects we learn as humans. Love and caring are also very much connected. You may have struggled all your life, feeling that your views did not matter, that you were less than other people, afraid of going into a room and feeling your opinion did not matter.

Students bring issues to the course and have often experienced mental health problems, such as anxiety and depression, themselves. What many people do not realise is that you can suffer emotionally and mentally without being mentally ill. Nurses and midwives do talk about times in their lives when they experienced and suffered with mental health problems. However, many talk about the effects of stigma and finding it hard to go back to work.

In practice

It is very upsetting to visit staff who are mentally and emotionally exhausted. It is very difficult to say, 'I'm so sorry things are so bad', then leave them there in the middle of it all. Mental health nurses are not being looked after and there is real hardship as fewer nurses are trying to cover care during staff absences (Ford, 2002; Sainsbury, 1998). Mental health nurses have a history of grin and bear it. It is deplorable given the plight of users, who are often unable to look after themselves and desperately need assistance with basic living.

Users cry and are desperate. Some hear voices and try to put on a brave face, but they have enormous care and compassion for nurses. They are people and can sense if a nurse is under pressure or not coping.

It may appear strange to have this kind of chapter in a book about becoming a mental health nurse, yet from a cursory glance at practice, it becomes self evident why nurses need to be concerned with these issues. We need to learn to take good care of ourselves in order to care for others effectively.

There are ways of looking after our mental health and everyone in mental health should be involved in protecting the rights of nurses in mental health care. This needs to come from effective government policy, resourcing policies, staff support groups, conditions of service, supportive supervision, team building away from the clinical area, teaching, and a proactive policy on human rights for all staff and users.

As individuals, we need to learn about our own mental health first before we care for others. We need to learn about how we cope and the issues we carry with us. An ongoing understanding of ourselves as people is important and students are often hungry for feedback. All those working in mental health need to appreciate issues concerned with coping and the journey people have to make, with or without help. The prevalence of mental health problems is a growing concern not only with the public, but also with health professionals. Health professionals are not immune to mental health problems, such as, depression or other emotional problems. Contrary to popular myths, there is no evidence to suggest that, because you are a mental health nurse, you will cope better or are immune.

Mental health nurses are human and have needs like anyone else. In the present climate, so much energy is expended in maintaining the service and much therapeutic time is lost in our work. You cannot appreciate the demands on a nurse's health until you see the demands in practice. We should have a vested interest in keeping staff healthy not just physically, but also mentally and emotionally. The demands are increasing for nurses in practice (Sainsbury, 1998).

The increasing demands on nurses

> 'Its eight thirty and I am due on duty at nine. I have butterflies in my stomach; just had an argument with my ten year old daughter and I know I am irritable but I have accepted this is part of being tired and stressed.'

> (Staff Nurse)

> 'Nurses aren't helped nearly enough to understand the sorts of feelings... the powerful processes that inevitably go on.'

> 'We tend to take our own mental and emotional health for granted. It is perhaps clear to experienced nurses that we may not take heed of the signs of occupational stress until sometimes it is too late.'

> 'Whatever is coming through the door... a broad spectrum... all and sundry... you cannot refuse... they're all under one roof... severe levels of anxiety, psychosis, high levels of depression, suicide... paranoia.'

> (Gijbels, 1995)

Stress and mental health nursing

Already, it is reported that nurses spend a shorter percentage of time with users or involved in therapeutic work (Sullivan, 1998). The reasons for this are numerous and should be of great concern to the profession. In summary, this is often due to lack of staffing, which reduces the nursing focus to maintaining safety, patrolling and containment, dealing with increased administrative work, poor working conditions, excessive occupancy levels, and staff that are often pressurised. Nurses are straddled between the demands of users versus the reality of resources in a sea of administration, an increasing number of new government policies, and a new mental health act.

In the middle of looking after other people and providing a variety of therapeutic interventions and care, the question remains as to whether nurses in mental healthcare really take care of themselves? Is there a way of being able to support mental health nurses in practice? Can we develop work practices that can support a nurse who experiences a mental health problem? What is clear is that the stress of being a mental health nurse, particularly in acute services, needs serious attention.

Stress in mental health nursing is receiving increasing attention (Handy, 1995; Jones, 1987; Laryea 2002; Paine, 1982; Thomas, 1997). The kindness, sensitivity and respect that nurses learn to give users and their families needs to be reflected back on nurses, who suffer psychologically and emotionally with stress in the course of their caring work.

Mental health nurses are men and women who have spent a minimum of three years in education to do the job they do. Many nurses have children and other responsibilities outside of work. They engage in further education and training after qualifying, and often work in difficult and volatile environments, such as, acute care, which are under-resourced (Sainsbury, 1998). Their work requires intelligent and decisive management and is practically, emotionally and psychologically intensive. The care burden is often high and the dependency level of users is significant. Abusive behaviour is sometimes experienced by staff in the course of their work. Recently, it has been shown that poor resources, changes in practice and stress can lead to interpersonal conflict and bullying behaviour in qualified nurses. Consequently, with respect to fitness to practice, nurses felt inadequately prepared in relation to care of people with enduring mental health problems (Laryea, 2002).

Student nurses, like qualified nurses, have lives outside their course of study that place demands on them. It is essential to grasp the reality of life for students, especially those with children, and to appreciate the need to integrate care structures for nurses as well as users. It is possible, as staffing resources are low, that staff members have increasing pressures to perform, so flexibility is diminished and this can place increasing burdens on individual nurses. In fact, nurses that are good at certain tasks may be left doing nothing but

that same task, which further reduces job satisfac\
increases psychological stress.

Currently in practice, nurses are facing the deman\
other professionals, users and their families, and if \ .e
number of nurses on duty dwindles, the work demands do
not change. This can cause an increased psychological burden,
feelings of failure and the using up of more and more energy.

Acute conditions

Conditions in acute wards are a cause for great concern
and appear to be worsening in the UK. According to one
report, patients only receive limited therapeutic input and
multidisciplinary care is absent for the majority. There is little
evidence of any involvement with psychologists and the
majority of admissions were unplanned 'emergency
admissions'. Indeed, users had little contact with other staff
apart from nurses and doctors (Sainsbury, 1998). It would
seem prudent to assess and address the health of nursing staff
given the enormous and relentless demands of care. This
chapter is aimed at students and other nurses and will
examine ways of encouraging them to look after their own
mental health.

In the present psychiatric machinery, nurses are almost
treated like workhorses; to deliver care wherever there is a
demand, irrespective of the working conditions or the state of
their own health.

> 'Administrative duties, responding to senior management and
> servicing other disciplines took priority over therapeutic
> activities. The clinical grade influenced the amount of time a
> nurse spent on administration, which resulted in the office
> becoming the focal point for a variety of interactions. You've got
> to work under high levels of pressure and tension, with less and
> less staff... you've got to be seen to be coping.'
>
> (Gijbels, 1995)

Working in mental health is different to many other
professions. It is demanding just by virtue of being in the
environment. Nurses have to be prepared to act, intervene,

communicate, and manage throughout a shift. Shift work is often antisocial, so nurses need to juggle their personal lives and, contrary to what many people think, have to be very loyal and supportive to colleagues.

This is incredible when weighed against the level of responsibility they have for others in their care, and the need to be caring and approachable while dealing with the demands of others. This includes other professionals who all think their requests should have priority. If you are in charge of a shift, it should not be presumed you have a skill mix that will compliment the demands of care on that particular shift. Furthermore, nurses may be off sick, there are emergency admissions, escort duties or continual demands from other areas that are short of staff.

Neither doctors nor medicine have all the answers in relation to looking after people's mental health. Although they may have compassion, the reality is that the conditions are not their responsibility.

The Medical Model

'These gods in white coats are not infallible.'

(Maynard, 2002)

It is evident that medicine continues to hold the power base in psychiatry. Some nurses are deceived by the thought that, because they can speak in a ward round and are on first name terms with consultants, their opinions are considered equal. Sadly they are not. Doctors still hold the larger power share as they have done throughout the medicalisation of madness. Of more concern is that psychiatry, as a role model, is significantly flawed and failing the development of humane care. Science is not just about knowledge, it is also about understanding. Understanding is perhaps one area psychiatry and nursing need to cultivate today. The medical model continues to focus on illness and, as a result, it is not addressing many of the social and caring issues. Most clinical approaches in psychiatry seem to bypass social problems and feelings, and very limited time is provide to encourage, instil hope or promote personal growth for users, or nurses. Much of the burden of understanding and caring is then left to nurses.

Nurses! Take care of yourselves

In order for nurses to take care of their physical and mental health, it is essential to acknowledge their rights as human beings, and this also needs to apply to users of mental health services. It seems strange that we need to remind services of the importance of valuing their workforce, particularly valuing nursing staff. The irony is that nurses represent caring, but are often viewed as the last people to be cared for. Perhaps a nurse is seen as a self-sufficient caring machine for others, as if all the caring they give is donated to some internal caring reserve. It is difficult to meet a nurse who is a patient on an acute ward without realising that the demands of the job and lack of support could have contributed to his/her predicament.

It is not surprising that nurses to suffer with mental health problems when you see what they have to cope with day in and day out. We should be extremely concerned about mental health nurses (Hiscott and Connop, 1990); there is a serious need to put in place a programme to safeguard their health and mental well-being. In some ways, the nursing ethos, like the admiration for Florence Nightingale, idealises the nurse as helper and healer with little consideration for the needs of nurses themselves. Such an ideal is completely at odds not only with physical health, but also with any appreciation or understanding of emotional or mental well-being.

Understanding life for student nurses requires us to dispense with much of the fantasy surrounding our view of student life. Being a student nurse is demanding emotionally, psychologically and physically. It requires structured support, a personal tutor, a clinical practice supervisor, and incredible stamina to survive in mental health settings. Here a student gives an account of a day in her life with the added responsibility of two young children.

Student life

5.45am	Alarm, Get children up
6.00am	Leave House to take boyfriend to work
7.00am	Get children ready for school
8.00am	Drop children at school
8.10am	Get ready myself
9.00am	At University
4.00pm	Leave University to go to shops
4.30pm	One hour study
5.45pm	Pick children up from after school club
6.30pm	Bath and feed children
7.30pm	Put them to bed, and from then on this is my time to do housework, study and sleep

The above indicates the high levels of stress that are compounded by virtue of being a full-time student with children. The student may not always be aware of the need to manage and plan, particularly around clinical placements. Even if the student has a partner, there may be considerable stress on their relationship.

A student who develops a mental health problem does not always feel able to seek help. Initially, the kind of support available is a student counselling service. Students may consider it to be a weakness to acknowledge psychological problems, in part because of fear of being withdrawn from the course. Such issues need to be managed sensitively and having a university policy helps. The following is a description of some distinctive features of change in a person, which may indicate they are suffering psychologically.

Tips for survival

Getting to know yourself

Fundamentally, to build confidence and self-esteem, you need to really appreciate who you are and be able to note down aspects of yourself that you are proud of. Self-esteem can be destroyed much easier than people think. It is not about qualifications, for you can have all these, but if your perception of yourself is still negative so, too, will be your self-esteem. It often requires coaching and support when the person has really learned maladaptive coping patterns as a result of prolonged stress. It is important to experience a workshop to appreciate that you are not alone in suffering from stress, anxiety or depression. To survive, you may need to try a new perspective that reflects the reality of your situation and can empower you to change. If you take a dance class, exercise class, yoga, or meditation, you cease to see yourself in the same way as you would in a class room. A major difference is that you are using your brain differently. In fact, if all you do is listen you will feel very tired. Each person has to find his/her own pace. It is essential that you explore relaxation for yourself. As mentioned earlier in the book, anxiety and depression are the most prevalent mental health problems today. You may have difficulty at the start as many people are not used to thinking positive thoughts about themselves.

The reality is that we have to work with ourselves to build the qualities we can use with others. For example, a person with negative thoughts may be easy to relate to, but needs someone who can help them restructure their thought patterns. To do this, you need to be confident in your own ability and skills. It is important to be able to identify your strengths, weaknesses, likes and dislikes.

It is not unusual for people to be burdened by negative self-concepts and body image. This often relates to how comfortable they are with being confronted or confronting other issues, body space, touch, topics they find difficult to discuss, disclosure to others, and perhaps how they feel about their own body. By recognising such issues, they can balance their health by investing in the areas on which they need to work. However, we are not always aware of how to take care of our emotional and psychological well-being. Regular exercise is one method of keeping fit, both mentally and physically (Morrissey, 1997).

Mental health nursing can cause feelings of mental and emotional tiredness. People talk of feeling drained. It is vital to manage the stress of working in an emotionally and psychologically intense atmosphere. Part of this requires each person to know and define his/her own limits. Help is often needed with developing this ability for, having learned to care, people often care too much, in some cases, to the point of suffering burnout. Nurses often feel responsible for each other. In ward cultures where there is a dependency on a team, morale is usually higher. All stress is not negative and it should be evident that achieving a goal requires investment and occasionally a side effect is stress or excitement.

Knowing your limits

It is important to know your limits emotionally and mentally. Many people carry and hold onto negative feelings that can make them feel very stressed. Crying is an outlet for some, which is a positive release. There is a need to learn how to find your emotional limits and how you can release tension.

Personality is an important factor, yet whatever your personality type, you need to work out ways to release your feelings, for example, by learning key breathing exercises, and then you can teach others. When tense, people are inclined to hold emotions in and when they relax, they release them. If a person feels under threat, the mind tends to hold on to emotions. It is essential to learn how to monitor your own body to tell it when to relax.

How do you cope with stress

Methods for coping with stress are individual. For nurses, there is a culture of 'I'm fine; honest'. It is a kind of emotional, macho culture. Nurses often need a complete break from the clinical area to be able to learn about relaxation. In reality, there is often nowhere to go for a break. In a strange way, nurses may be unable to practice what they preach. Relaxation alone will not always de-stress a person. People need to talk and feel they are being listened to. Groups are a useful way of talking through and sharing issues. There needs to be space to complain and be constructive. The way a ward is managed is, of course, part of this. If the ward is short staffed, it is not necessarily true that staff will be significantly more stressed. It really depends on their workload and their perception of stress. In busy acute wards, being under staffed is a critical situation. Nurses can burn out quickly. This is serious and means that the person's emotional and mental health has been significantly affected as a result of working conditions. This is often very upsetting for colleagues and needs much support.

Such situations need more than a few relaxation classes. The care of a person with burnout needs very significant yet sensitive consideration. On top of feeling redundant, the person needs to be cared for. The hospital or trust needs to take some responsibility for the situation in which such professionals find themselves; it is essential that he/she is not left to self-care and a partnership is required. There needs to be a system in place that takes better care of nurses in practice.

Management needs to be about caring for nurses in practice. This can be achieved by a regular review of the staff's health, and should include reviews of mental and emotional health. An environment needs to be provided where nurses can go on breaks that are designed for relaxation. If nurses do not take breaks, this is not always their fault; it might be that we need to address the work culture. A number of other issues also need addressing. Questions to be explored are how easy or difficult do you find it to ask for help and what strategy needs to be in place to help you survive as a student. Social support is necessary for healthy relationships with others, as is having a buddy system for students, so that they can share their day-to-day feelings with another student on the same journey. This can act as a stress shield.

Managing time is a vital skill for everyone, and it is important to get to grips with this issue, particularly if you have a family. Having a structure and a clear focus can reduce and make the path clearer. You will need to explore own ways of combatting stress, but exercise or other activities are a good start. Peace and quiet are often lacking, but are important for those working in the caring profession. A change of environment is very useful in helping students to relax.

No doubt changes as a person will occur during the process of becoming a mental health nurse, and you can manage how you are adapting. It is important not to leave individuals totally responsible for looking after their own mental health, but some responsibility for self care is essential. Often, those refusing help are the ones who need it most. Can nurses practice what they preach?

Practice what you preach

Stress in nursing is not a new concept; yet, on acute wards and in other mental health settings, it is evident that we need to learn to take care of ourselves for no-one else will (Dewe, 1987; Norcross *et al*, 2000). It seems absurd how many doctors and nurses spend time advising patients to cut down on smoking and drinking to enhance their health, when they, too, could benefit from the same advice. This is also the case in relation to mental health. Most mental health promotion literature seems to give a contradictory health stance (Becker, 1993; Evans, 1988). Promoting health needs not only to concentrate on empirical research, but also to be grounded in reality. If this is not the case, it seems unlikely that a sense of proportion and balance will be established for everyday living. Much of psychiatry continues to be concerned with medication and much of the current care practices do little to empower users or nurses. **More importantly, this is not the way nurses are trained to care**.

One of the most astonishing aspects of being a nurse is that it seems there is little caring or support available to nurses. Nurses deliver wherever there is a need and there is no real model of how it should be, how many hours of work, at what intensity, breaks, the need for careful support, such as away days, etc. Stress is synonymous with nursing (Laryea,

2002). Mental health problems among nurses are much more common than you might think; survival of the fittest is the norm and burnout is common.

Nurses are beginning to recognise the need to establish better ways of living not just to promote mental health, but to cope with demands and reduce them. Self-help is not just a resource for users (Norcross *et al*, 2000), and making people aware of their mental health needs is useless, unless their working conditions and workload are reviewed and changed. This alone can bring a sense of control, an ability to make real choices and help to re-establish positive habits.

Nurses are real people with needs like anyone else. They are working in incredibly stressful environments in acute care, and often work on wards where there are staff shortages. As a consequence, they can have little time for establishing opportunities that create and sustain mental health for themselves. Mental health nurses work with users, but who looks after nurses? We live in an era where the adverts tell us to look after our body. We spend a fortune on beauty products, yet mental health is frequently ignored? The most extraordinary facet of being a mental health nurse is the lack of appreciation concerning our own mental health. It is time for nurses to take good care of their own emotional and mental well-being. If we are not careful, it will be the sick tending the sick and, in some areas, that is already the case.

Useful Web Addresses in Mental Health

Help-Direct Database

http://www.hfht.org/databases/helpdirect.htm
Help-Direct is a comprehensive, searchable database of self-help and support groups, and organizations covering the whole of the UK, and available to the public on the Internet. Information is continually updated, with local groups being added for many areas. GP, pharmacy, optical and dentist information is also available for some areas. If you want to include information on this database, contact the editing

team: editors@hfht.org. Future development of this Website to explore users wants and needs.

NHS Direct

http://www.nhsdirect.nhs.uk

This site gives information about many health matters and the section is particularly informative in relation to mental health.

National Electronic Library for Mental Health

http://www.nelh.nhs.uk/

The NeLMH is one of the first virtual branch libraries of the National Electronic Library for Health strategy. The NeLMH is also one of the main areas of focus for the Mental Health Information Strategy announced in the National Service Framework for Mental Health.

References

Becker MH (1993) A medical sociologist looks at health promotion. *J Health Social Behav* **34**(March): 11–16

Blacker C, Clare A (1987) Depressive disorder in primary care. *Br J Psychiatry* **150**: 737–51

Dewe PJ (1987) Identifying strategies nurses use to cope with work stress. *W J Nurs Res* **12**: 489–97

Evans RI (1988) Health promotion science or ideology? *Health Psychol* **7**(3): 203–19

Ford R (2002) Opinion (Personal opinion on government policy for mental health services, emphasizing the need to value nurses working in acute patient care). *Ment Health Pract* **5**(9): 26

Gijbels H (1995) Mental health nursing skills in an acute admission environment: perceptions of mental health nurses and other professionals. *J Adv Nurs* **21**(3): 460–65

Handy J (1995) Stress in mental health nursing: a socio-political analysis. Cited in: Carson J *et al. Stress and Coping in Mental Health Nursing*. Chapman and Hall, London

Hiscott RD, Connop PJ (1990) The health and well-being of mental health professionals. *Can J Pub Health* **81**(6): 422–26

Jones JG (1987) Stress in psychiatric nursing. In: Paine R, Firth-Cozens R, eds. *Stress in Health Professionals*. John Wiley and Sons, Chichester

Laryea T (2002) Perceptions of occupational stress in psychiatric/mental health nurses. Working with people with enduring mental illnesses in a rehabilitation setting. De Montfort University Leicester: unpublished MA Thesis

Maynard A (2002) These gods are not infallible. *Daily Mail*, Friday November 1: 17

Merrell KW (2001) *Helping Students Overcome Depression and Anxiety: A Practical Guide*. The Guilford Press, New York: 231

Morrissey M (1997) Mood enhancement and anxiety reduction using physical exercise in a clinical sample. *Int J Psychiatr Nurs Res* **3**(2): 336–44

Norcross JC, Santrock JW, Campbell LF, Smith TP, Sommer R, Zuckerman EL (2000) Authoritative guide to self-help

resources in mental health.
http://biomed.niss.ac.uk/ovidweb/ovidweb.cgi

Paine WS (1982) *Job Stress and Burnout Stress: Research, Theory and Intervention Perspectives*. Sage, London

Sainsbury (1998) *Briefing Paper 4: Acute problems: A Survey of the Quality of Care in Acute Psychiatric Wards*. Sainsbury Centre for Mental Health, London

Sullivan P (1998) Therapeutic interaction in mental health nursing. *Nurs Stand* **12**(45): 39–42

Thomas B (1997) Management strategies to tackle stress in mental health nursing. *Ment Health Care* **1**(1): 15–17

8

Tending the human heart: A Mother's Story

'We live in a society that demands a quick fix to life's problems yet there is so much more to helping someone than getting their medication right.'

(Morrissey, 1999)

This chapter is devoted to the courage of a parent, partner, friend or sibling who care for a family member with a mental health problem. It is impossible to convey the immense respect, love, patience, strength and financial resources that are required to be a carer in today's society. Nurses can describe many stories about the amazing courage of users and their relatives. In order to provide an appreciation of the reality of having a mental health problem, the story of one mother and her son will be outlined. Mental health needs to be very much about feelings and caring, as there is no miracle cure for individuals who are labelled as schizophrenic. Of more importance is supporting carers and families and providing early intervention where possible. Quality of life is a prime factor, so the individual needs to have planned care, which must include education and meaningful skills for living. Nurses need to be in a position to provide support so they can inform and understand the needs of carers as well as users.

Having a mental health problem, such as schizophrenia or bi-polar affective disorder, can turn a person into a shadow of his/her former self. The consequences of a mental health problem can be devastating not just for the person, but for partners, parents and other family members. The fact that people have to get on with their lives, even though they have a mental health problem, is often forgotten. The following story of a mother's experience of caring for her son, diagnosed with schizophrenia, illustrates that caring for the mind also involves tending the human heart.

A Mother's Story

'My family and I are still going through heartache over the care of my son. Andy was born in 1973 and had a traumatic birth, which was upsetting for me and my husband. I was scared, like all mothers, and also felt terrible anxiety about the baby for a long time after the birth. He took an unusually long time to learn to speak.

He started prep school at three, where he was a sensitive and fun-loving child. He was very well-behaved and much liked. When he was six, he started at primary school, where other mothers noted that Andy was highly sensitive and found it difficult to mix with girls. Academically, he did very well and went on to pass his eleven-plus examination.

He went to grammar school where he met his now best friend, Elliott, and his sensitivity was again remarked on by the teachers. During his teenage years, he was a joy to be around. He was great company, well read and full of compassion. We had wonderful conversations, lots of laughter. He had several hobbies, mainly music and photography, and formed a band with his friends. He passed 10 O-levels (GCSEs) and four A-levels.

During his year out before university, he took a City and Guilds diploma in photography and arranged a trip to India. On his return in 1992 he was full of enthusiasm about starting his degree in London. He began his course in October. Within days, his grandfather died.

This had a profound effect on Andy over the next few months. He became involved with people who took advantage of his generosity and declining mental state. Three months into the degree course he came home and stayed longer than his holidays, as he did not feel well. I never suspected a mental health problem.

In February 1993, he contracted measles and throughout the year marked changes in his personality and behaviour took place. He became very withdrawn and hypersensitive; conversations were frequently scrambled and disjointed. My husband and I were very distressed by this, but continued to deny our dawning realisation that something was terribly wrong. His first admission to a psychiatric hospital broke my heart. I cried almost all the time. I found it unbearable to see my lovely son sitting in a psychiatric ward clearly suffering. I felt helpless. My husband, son and daughter were quietly devastated.

I was shocked by the coldness and harshness of the environment and the decline of my son in front of my eyes. I knew nothing about schizophrenia until my son was diagnosed, which took a couple of years. There were many times when I felt completely deserted and unsupported. I was shocked at the lack of qualified nurses on Andy's ward.

Some staff were very helpful.

I was delighted with those who were intelligent and practical about the problems I had with Andy when he was in hospital. But his GP lacked any deep understanding of schizophrenia, frequently reminding me how busy he was.

Recently, Andy was placed under a section of the Mental Health Act, which again caused me tears, constant worry and guilt. When he was very unwell, I was asked not to visit. Relationships at home had become difficult and sensitive and I doubt that the staff had any idea of the juggling I had to do as a mother, carer, wife and professional person.

Several times senior staff spoke about my son as though he were not a real, intelligent person capable of making decisions.

Over the past few years I have lived in the world of mental health care. I have had to learn to grit my teeth and bite my lip in order to get good care for Andy. I have feared upsetting or challenging the staff in case it affected his care. Some staff saw me as trouble because I demanded the best care for my son. Whatever happens, I know I am the one he counts on. I worry about what would happen if I were not around. One day I sat in my car talking with a friend and I watched a young man pass by just like Andy. I cried and realised how I wished Andy could be as he used to be. I still remember the kind, compassionate and well-mannered young man. When you love someone, you want them to be happy. I am sitting here with my son trying to face things in a smoke-filled hospital day room. I can't pretend things are all right.

Now that I know more, I realise how brave Andy is and how tolerant he is of ignorant people. I always feel lonely as I leave him during one of his spells in hospital, yet I am fearful when he is at home. Increasingly, I just have to get on with things, as Andy has to.

I wonder who will take care of him should anything happen to me or my husband. We have had so many arguments at home and his brother and sister have both wished he would disappear. I have blamed myself, thinking I was my fault. My husband is unable to cope with the demands of continuous support and care. It is during the quiet times I really despair about mental health services.

Even though many people are against medication, I know it is necessary to help calm Andy and restore him to his former self He suffers dreadfully both psychologically and emotionally and, of course, I would go to the ends of the earth, like any loving parent, to comfort him. But the worst part of schizophrenia is that at times the person is almost impossible to comfort. This often means the person is unable to engage in close, intimate human contact. Andy has lost all his friends apart from Elliott. This upsets me and him, as he really loved them. But with each hospital admission, another friend left.

The most negative effect of schizophrenia is the fact that it keeps coming back. Such episodes are relentless, cruel and strip the special qualities that make Andy who he is and the son I dearly love. I must admit that I have been scared of my own son at times, but the love I have has made me strong, a survivor and at times more knowledgeable than those dispensing care'.

Reflection on what we do

People affected by mental health problems have very human needs—love, compassion, warmth, understanding—but these are often marginalised by the concepts and language of modern psychology and psychiatry. In essence, mental health nursing should be an offering of humanity before being a branch of medicine. There are other problems: the dearth of qualified staff, lack of suitable therapeutic environments to foster feelings of safety and emotional warmth, poor support, education and information and fear about future care provision.

The job of a mental health nurse is taxing and skilled, compromised by current work practices and the demands of poorly resources services. They need resources to allow them to care in ways other than diagnosing, medicating and monitoring (Barker *et al*, 1997). The enduring nature of mental health problems, such as schizophrenia, and their effects on families, must be recognised. Our society demands a quick fix to life's problems, yet there is more to helping someone than getting the medication right. Nurses need time and space for therapeutic interventions with clients.

Academic debate over what exactly constitutes mental health does little for poorly resourced services and demoralised professionals. The practical aspects of caring tend to be undervalued (Bradshaw, 1998). One of the magical aspects of being a mental health nurse is helping reduce a person's distress, if only for a moment.

What many psychotherapists and academics fail to grasp is that the healing process needs to be holistic, dynamic and sometimes diverse. It can be so hard to reach some people and this is when you really need the skills of nurses. When individuals require help and comfort with enduring mental health problems, they frequently need determined and sustained intervention (Gamble and Brennan, 2001).

Loss is a pervasive feeling for users and often a great shared sense of sadness for nurses. Mental health nurses often have incredible resourcefulness and an amazing sense of humour in spite of much adversity. It is important to value the great contribution a caring mental health nurse can make in the life of another person. The nursing profession must nurture not only knowledge, but also human qualities, such as love, compassion and understanding—an important part of mental health care. There are many treatments for mental health problems, but most of them bypass human emotions and the human spirit. Sometimes, a piece of music or a song can comfort us and comfort needs to be an important part of caring. The words of the song Bridge Over Troubled Waters was originally sung by Simon and Garfunkel, but was recorded by Eva Cassidy on her album Live at Blues Alley. Eva was an incredibly shy, sensitive, loving and gifted person and her interpretation of this song echoes values that can touch each of us. Mental health nursing is about friendship and support and nurses are a big part of any support bridge. In the end, as oxygen is to the brain, so is friendship and social support to the human heart. Kindness and strength remain important qualities in supporting individuals with a mental health problem, as does the courage to face their diagnosis. The importance of such qualities is best put by Princess Diana's favourite quote.

'Life is like froth and bubbles, but two things stand out—kindness in someone else's troubles and courage in your own'.

Friendship and caring remain important in supporting a person with a mental health problem, like schizophrenia. At times, the person may be unaware of his or her own needs. Such vulnerability is what many parents are acutely aware of. It is such a hard reality for a caring mother to see the deterioration of a person she loves and cherishes.There is a real need to build bridges of care. More than ever, we need to be united in care whatever our professional background, to relieve emotional and psychological suffering in the knowledge and truth that cures continue to remain elusive. I leave you with the words of a song, which expresses so much about the value of hope instilled by friendship. This kind of medicine is now perhaps not just powerful, but increasingly rare.

Bridge over troubled water

When you're weary, feeling small
When tears are in your eyes, I will dry them all.
I'm on your side.
Oh when times get rough

And friends just can't be found
Like a bridge over troubled water
I will lay me down.
Like a bridge over troubled water
I will lay me down.
When you're down and out,
When you're on the street
When evening falls so hard
I will comfort you.
I'll take your part.
Oh when darkness comes
And pain is all around
Like a bridge over troubled water
I will lay me down
Like a bridge over troubled water
I will lay me down.
Sail on silver girl, sail on by,
Your time has come to shine
All your dreams are on their way
See how they shine
Oh if you need a friend
I'm sailing right behind
Like a bridge over troubled water
I will ease your mind
Like a bridge over troubled water
I will ease your mind.

Eva Cassidy (1963–1996)

References

Barker P, *et al* (1997) The human science basis of psychiatric nursing: theory and practice. *J Adv Nurs* **25**(4): 660–67

Bradshaw A (1998) Charting some challenges in the art and science of nursing. *Lancet* **351**(9100): 438–40

Cassidy E (1996) *Live at Blues Alley*. Hotrecords, Brighton, UK

Gamble C, Brennan G (2001) *Working with Serious Mental Illness: A Manual for Clinical Practice*. Balliere Tindall, Harcourt Publishers Limited, London

Morrissey M (1999) Fellow Feelings…a mother's story of caring for her son, diagnosed with schizophrenia. *Nurs Times* **95**(21): 38–39

Index

Index

Index